IS IT LEAKY GUT
OR
LEAKY GUT SYNDROME?

Clean Gut, Allergies, Fatty Liver, Autoimmune Diseases, Fibromyalgia, Multiple Sclerosis, Autism, Psoriasis, Diabetes, Cancer, Parkinson's, Thyroiditis, & More

Anil Minocha MD

Professor of Medicine
Certified, Physician Nutrition Support Specialist
Fellow, American College of Physicians
Fellow, American College of Gastroenterology
Fellow, American Gastroenterological Association

Copyright

Disclaimer: The publisher has put forth its best efforts in preparing and arranging this book. The information provided herein by the author is provided "as is" and you read and use this information at your own risk. The publisher and author disclaim any liabilities for any loss of profit or commercial or personal damages resulting from the use of the information contained in this book.

This work is meant for informational use only and by no means represents recommendations for diagnosis or treatment of any disorder for any reader. Neither the publisher nor the author is engaged in rendering medical advice or services to any individual reader. Nothing in this book is intended to be a substitute for consultation with a licensed physician. All matters of health require medical supervision. While intestinal permeability or leaky gut has been well documented in medical literature, the concept of leaky gut syndrome is considered controversial in some quarters. The book is meant to provide you with information so you may make your own decisions. Only your licensed medical provider can determine what remedies are in the best interest of your health and what to do about your illness. Never implement any health information from a book without discussing it with your physician.

The procedures, treatments, and practices described in this book should be implemented only by a licensed physician and only in a manner consistent with the professional standards set for the circumstances that apply in each specific situation. Neither the publisher nor the author is responsible for your specific health or allergy needs that may require medical attention. The author, editor, and publisher cannot accept responsibility for errors, exclusions, or the outcome of the application of the material presented herein. There is no expressed or implied warranty of this book or the information imparted by it.

Neither the publisher nor the author has financial interest in the pharmaceuticals, over-the-counter medications including supplements, or any medical equipment mentioned in this book.

PREFACE

I think we ought always to entertain our opinions with some measure of doubt. I shouldn't wish people dogmatically to believe any philosophy, not even mine.
—Bertrand Russell

Medicine is an art, not a science, and our already vast knowledge is increasing exponentially. This book fulfills the need for a quick, concise source of practical information, allowing the reader to better understand the concept of leaky gut and be a better-informed consumer of health information, especially during a visit to the physician.

To achieve the goal of providing a condensed version of the state of knowledge for a broad audience, I have presented the current state of literature as well as controversial positions. As in most cases of medical science, everyone has an opinion. Knowledge that was deemed to be an indisputable fact only a few years ago may now be cast away as rubbish. Just take an example of fats, including saturated fats, which are no longer considered to be as bad as was taught and practiced for decades! Bacteria in the stomach have now been confirmed to be a major cause of ulcers, even though the concept of infection-causing ulcers had been dismissed for decades as an old wives' tale.

I am of the opinion that our gut plays a critical role in health and sickness. This is not a new concept. Hippocrates thought of the same thing thousands of years ago when he stated, "All diseases begin in the gut."

Digestive and immune processes, including disordered gut structure and function as well as gut psychology, play a critical role not just in GI illnesses, but they have also been implicated in neurobehavioral disorders (autism, ADHD, OCD), chronic pain syndromes (fibromyalgia, chronic fatigue syndrome, restless leg syndrome, temporo-mandibular joint disorder [TMJD], migraine headache), autoimmune conditions (rheumatoid arthritis, ankylosing spondylitis), and skin disorders like allergies, skin eczema, acne, and psoriasis. The gut has a brain of its own, and the term "gut psychology" has been used to describe the role of the gut in anxiety and depression.

Evidence indicates that the digestion connection to your overall health is real. The use of terms like perfect digestion (Dr. Deepak Chopra), digestive wellness (Dr. Elizabeth Lipski), healthy digestion (Dr. Lindsey Berkson), and gutbliss (Dr. Robynne Chutkan) highlights the importance of our gut in overall health. Books on the integrative approach to treatment of chronic diseases, e.g. "Integrative Gastroenterology", a part of Andrew Weil Integrative Medicine series and edited by Gerard Mullin, MD a renowned gastroenterologist from the Johns Hopkins School of Medicine in Baltimore, MD, are becoming increasingly popular. By the way, I was privileged to contribute a chapter to Dr. Mullin's book.

I have at times in this book, sacrificed finer detail and nuances for the sake of brevity and clarity. This book should not be used to make a diagnosis or initiate any treatment. All illness requires medical supervision by a licensed physician. And yes, I have had my own health challenges in life. That is all the more reason for me to share what I have learned both professionally and personally over the years.

Knowledge is broad-based, and each person is unique. It is critical that no one adopt any changes based on this book or for that matter any other book without discussing them with a physician.

I wish all the readers a happy and healthy life.

FOREWORD

Leaky Gut Syndrome is an issue of importance to us all, whether you've heard of it or not. The lining of your small intestine has a big job even though it's only one cell thick -- to allow in nutrients while keeping unwanted microbes, chemicals, molds, and large food molecules out of your bloodstream. When this fails, we have leaky gut, or more correctly, increased intestinal permeability. While not a disease in and of itself, it underlies autoimmune conditions such as celiac disease, rheumatoid arthritis, multiple sclerosis, and Parkinson's disease.

Leaky gut also plays a role in obesity, mood disorders, how well your hormones work, asthma, eczema, psoriasis, and pain because when we have a leaky gut, we also have leaky skin, leaky lungs, and leaky brains!

Digestion is the river of life. When it fails to flow properly, our cells don't get the nourishment they need to keep us feeling optimally.

Dr. Minocha has written a comprehensive, yet concise, book on Leaky Gut Syndrome. He describes what it is, what contributes to it, and how it affects us in so many ways. One of the great strengths of this book is the research he has done on how leaky gut underlies such a wide variety of diseases and conditions, ranging from liver disease to neurological conditions, heart disease, arthritis, and diabetes. He takes complex interactions and simplifies them in descriptions and drawings so that anyone can understand them and then he gives you the tools to help heal.

So if you don't feel exactly the way you'd like to feel, it just may be that this book helps you find your path to well-being.

Elizabeth Lipski, PhD, CCN, CNS

Author of *Digestive Wellness, Digestive Wellness for Children*, and *Digestion Connection*

Director of Academic Development of the Nutrition Programs at Maryland University of Integrative Health

TABLE OF CONTENTS

Copyright ii

Preface v

Foreword...vii

SECTION I: Leaky Gut or Leaky Gut Syndrome... xix

Chapter 1: Chronic Illnesses are Widespread 1

Multitude of Disorders: An Accident or a Coincidence? 1

Who Should Read this Book?...2

Dr. M's Goals for the Reader 4

Presentation of a Holistic Approach to Healing Disordered Gut.....4

Barriology: the New Scientific Field Focusing on Gut Barrier........5

What has changed or not changed in recent times?........................6

Why Does Disease Not Occur in Everyone Under Similar
Circumstances?...7

Potential scenarios 8

Chapter 2: Healthy Gut 11

Healthy Dynamic Balance of 5 Factors is a Prerequisite for a
Healthy Gut/Body 12

The Gut is a Dynamic Stage with Ongoing Dialogue or Cross-talk
Among Actors 13

Chapter 3: Intestinal Barrier...15

Barrage of Toxic Insults 15

A single layer of gut cells separates body from poop................16

Composition of intestinal barrier..18

What is a Biofilm? 18

Chapter 4: The Gut: Is it Leaky or Not Leaky? 21

Passage of Substances Across the Gut Wall....................................22

Two pathways are involved 22

Pores in the gut 22

Tight Junctions 24

Gut wall is like chain fence...24

Tight junctions are picky...25

Chapter 5: Factors Affecting Gut Leakiness 27

Effect of Changes in Intestinal Bacteria 28

Human factors 29

Environmental factors 29

Dietary factors..30

Gut leakiness and food processing 31

Water and fluid intake..31

Food components affecting tight junctions in the gut wall 32

Potential Toxins That We Consume................................32

Gliadin/gluten..32

Food surfactants 33

Alcohol...33

Therapeutic states 34

Miscellaneous Factors Affecting Gut Permeability or Leakiness 35

Normal factors in a healthy person 35

Abnormal factors..36

Chapter 6: Leaky Gut Barrier 39

Inflammation and Leaky Barrier are Inter-linked........39

Inflammatory bowel disease...40

Graft versus host disease 40

Celiac sprue..40

Effects of Leaky Gut 40

Healthy gut 41

Unhealthy gut 41

Is Leaky Gut or Increased Intestinal Permeability a Disease?.........41
   Potential consequences of leaky gut in early life......................41
Chapter 7: How Does Leaky Gut Cause its Effects.........................43
  What Happens in Leaky Gut...43
   Tight junctions open..43
   Chain reaction of translocation 43
   Outburst of reactive oxygen species 44
   Oxidative burst in an attack mode...45
   Oxidative burst in leaky gut 46
   Oxidative burst can even be life-threatening.........................46
   Action 46
   Leaky gut impairs gut detoxification mechanisms.................47
  Biological Evidence of Leaky Gut..47
   Leaky gut and malabsorption can co-exist 48

SECTION II: Diseases Associated with Leaky Gut..51

Chapter 8: Leaky Gut Syndrome 53
  What Came First: Leaky Gut or the Disease...............................53
  Unhealthy Gene for Leaky Gut Does Not Equal Disease.............54
   Genes may be silent, over- or underactive.............................54
Chapter 9: Autoimmune Diseases of Various Kinds May Occur ...57
  Features of Autoimmune Disease...58
  Role of Testing for Leaky Gut..58
Chapter 10: Select Listing of Diseases Linked to Leaky Gut.........61
  Interpreting Tests for Leaky Gut..61
   GI diseases 61
   Endocrine diseases...62
   Allergic disorders 62
   Bacterial infections 62

Viral infections 62

Skin diseases 62

Liver diseases 63

Rheumatological diseases 63

Vascular (blood vessels) system 63

Neuro-psycho-behavioral dysfunction 63

Neurological disorders 64

Miscellaneous 64

Chapter 11: GI Diseases 67

Irritable Bowel Syndrome 67

Functional disorder 67

Evidence for leaky gut 67

Leaky gut and immune system 68

Celiac Disease 68

How does it occur? 69

Improved gut leakiness as a marker of recovery on a gluten-free diet 70

Inflammatory Bowel Disease 70

Evidence for leaky gut 71

Presence of leaky gut may predict relapse 71

NSAID-Induced Gut Disease (NSAID Enteropathy) 72

Chapter 12: Liver Diseases 75

Liver Cirrhosis 75

Hepatic Encephalopathy (Brain Dysfunction of Liver Disease) 76

Alcoholic Liver Disease 76

Fatty Liver Disease 77

Primary Biliary Cirrhosis (PBC) 77

Intrahepatic Cholestasis of Pregnancy 77

Chapter 13: Endocrine Diseases 81

    Diabetes Mellitus 81

        Factors involved 81

        Animal studies...81

        Human data 83

    Autoimmune Thyroiditis...83

        Gut inflammation 83

        Evidence for leaky gut 84

Chapter 14: Can't Lose Weight? It's Not Just Wheat Belly! 85

    Altered Gut Bacteria...85

        Intestinal leakiness..85

        Differences in energy harvest 86

    Role of Early Life Events 86

        Potential interventions...86

Chapter 15: Joint Diseases 89

    Arthritis 89

        Evidence for leaky gut 89

        Effect of fasting 90

        Role of probiotics 90

    Ankylosing Spondylitis..90

        Evidence for leaky gut 90

        Why is there discrepancy in test results sometimes 91

SECTION III: Neuro-behavioral Dysfunction 93

Chapter 16: Autism..95

    Leaky Gut Explains Brain Dysfunction 95

        Data implicating leaky gut in autism 96

        Further evidence for leaky gut in autism................................96

        Systems model for regressive autism 97

Effect of increased propionic acid 97

Therapeutic evidence 97

Multi-dimensional strategy is required................................98

Chapter 17: Psychiatric Disorders 101

Depression 101

Human data 102

More on stress and intestinal bacteria 104

Melancholic microbes versus probiotics..........................104

Gut disorder may underlie co-existing depression and
heart disease 105

Unhealthy gut may underlie PTSD too! 105

Schizophrenia..106

Schizophrenia and celiac disease 106

Effect of gluten and cow's milk.......................................106

Chapter 18: Neuro-degenerative Diseases 109

Multiple Sclerosis 109

MS and gut bacteria 110

Tight junctions in MS 110

Gluten sensitivity 110

Role of gluten free diet 111

Parkinson's Disease 111

Lewy bodies of Parkinson's are also seen in gut 111

Leaky gut in Parkinson's disease......................................112

SECTION IV: Chronic Pain Disorders 115

Chapter 19: Distinct Pain Disorders or One Syndrome?.............117

Are Different Diagnosis an Artificial Separation? 118

Diagnosis based on specialist seen....................................118

Unifying factors for the chronic pain disorders 118

Similarity in factors related to chronic pain disorders 119
Unified Framework to Explain the Underlying Process 119

Chapter 20: Chronic Fatigue Syndrome 123
Multiple Associations of CFS 123
Mechanism of disease 123
Increased antibodies against gut bacteria 124
Antibodies against cow proteins 124

Chapter 21: Fibromyalgia 127
Leaky Gut in Fibromyalgia 127
Co-occurrence with SIBO 127
Effect of gluten free diet 128

Chapter 22: Abdominal Migraine 129
Recurrent Abdominal Pain and Migraine 129
Features of abdominal migraine 130

**Chapter 23: Complex Regional Pain Syndrome or
Reflex Sympathetic Dystrophy 133**
CRPS/RSD is Known by Various Names 133
Evidence for leak gut 133
Altered intestinal bacterial patterns 134

**Section V: Tentacles of Gut Dysfunction:
A Potpourri 135**
Chapter 24: Food Allergies and Asthma 137
Food Allergies 137
Steps in causation 137
Food allergies and leaky gut 138
New allergies after liver transplantation 138
Eosinophilic esophagitis 138

Asthma...139
   Interaction of gene-environment 139
   Role of gut bacteria 140
   Leaky gut and asthma.......................................140
   Asthma and gut immune system..........................140

Chapter 25: Skin Diseases **143**
   Gut-Skin-Immune-Brain Axis 143
   Skin Eczema or Atopic Dermatitis..........................144
   Acne..145
   Psoriasis...145
   Rosacea 146
   Urticaria 147

Chapter 26: Miscellaneous **149**
   Cancer...149
   HIV Infection and AIDS...................................150
   Aging-associated Dementia 150
   Congestive Heart Failure (CHF) 151

SECTION VI: What if You Suspect Leaky Gut...... 153

Chapter 27: Testing for Leaky Gut.............................155
   Sugar-based Tests...156
      Lactulose-mannitol test 156
   Indirect Tests 156
   Screening for Leaky Gut....................................156
      Should we test and screen?..............................156
      Potential candidates for screening.....................157
      A successful story.......................................157

Chapter 28: How to Prevent and Strengthen Leaky Gut Barrier ..159
   Leaky Gut Prevention.......................................160
   Using Supplements to Strengthen Leaky Gut 160

Probiotics Enhance Barrier Function 160

Treatment Based on Underlying Factors 161

Example of treatment of small intestinal
bacterial overgrowth 161

Strengthen barrier, treat leaky gut! 162

Nutritional Approach to Strengthen Barrier 164

Role of Pharmaceutical Industry 165

Chapter 29: Probiotics and Prebiotics for Leaky Gut 167

All Probiotics are *Not* Created Similar or Equal 168

Examples of probiotics that strengthen gut barrier 168

Study the fine print on the label wisely 168

Type and number of bacteria is important 169

There is strength in numbers 169

Third party certifications 169

Importance of Prebiotics 169

Fiber-free diet makes gut leaky 170

Examples of naturally delicious prebiotics 170

Chapter 30: Holistic Gut-Venture Beyond Leaky Barrier 173

The Big Picture 173

One size does not fit all 173

Complex situations require comprehensive strategy 174

Dr. M's Closing Thoughts 175

The Choice is yours 175

A personal note from Dr. Minocha 177

Dedication 179

Praise for "Dr. M's Seven-X Plan for Digestive Health" 180

Other Books by Dr. Minocha 181

SECTION I

Leaky Gut or Leaky Gut Syndrome

CHAPTER 1

Chronic Illnesses are Widespread

KEY POINTS

- There has been an increase in a variety of poorly explained illnesses in recent decades.

- Disordered gut, especially leaky gut, may explain many of these illnesses that tend to co-occur in many subjects.

- The science of study of intestinal barrier is in its infancy and has been dubbed as barriology.

Do not fear to be eccentric in opinion, for every opinion now accepted was once eccentric.
—Bertrand Russell

MULTITUDE OF DISORDERS: AN ACCIDENT OR A COINCIDENCE?

There has been a rising tide of chronic unexplained illnesses in recent decades including chronic bowel problems, difficult to treat skin diseases like eczema and psoriasis, neurobehavioral issues like autism and ADHD, as well as chronic pain syndromes like fibromyalgia, chronic pain syndrome, and migraine.

It is common for an individual to suffer from more than one disorder suggesting a common underlying theme. Could that underlying theme be leaky gut?

1

Our Modern Life

- Almost one in three has a digestive system disorder
- Over 60 million show signs of or have subclinical evidence of autoimmune disease
- 125 million have chronic disease

•Is this is an accident?
•Is this a coincidence?

WHO SHOULD READ THIS BOOK?

Medical science is in a state of continued flux. If history is any guide, most of the things we practice today are likely to be outdated within two to three decades. It is not surprising that many patients don't get answers or relief from their problems since they are only taking "outdated treatments of the future."

Medical practitioners tend to be inflexible and frequently tied down with what they learned in medical school, what they learn at the occasional conferences they go to, or the drug sales representatives that come and visit them.

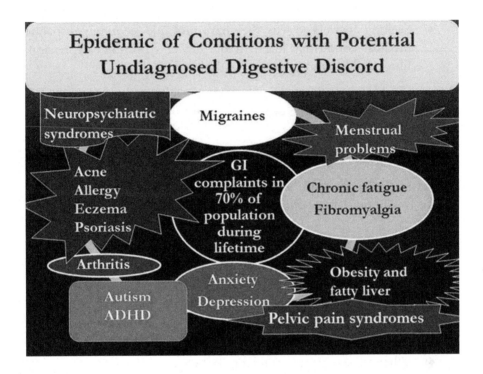

Hippocrates aptly stated, *"All diseases begin in the gut."*

This book is targeted at readers who wish to gain insights into the rapidly advancing field of intestinal barrier:

- Suffering from difficult to treat chronic gastrointestinal disorders.

- Suffering from obesity and unable to figure out why they are unable to control weight despite dieting.

- Believe that leaky gut may be involved in their condition: difficult to manage skin diseases like psoriasis, acne, and skin eczema.

- Seeking alternate options for their unanswerable neurobehavioral and pain syndromes like autism, fibromyalgia, chronic fatigue syndrome, and depression.

- Seeking answers to why they have multiple seemingly disparate medical conditions like irritable bowel syndrome, depression, fibromyalgia, and migraine headaches.

- Unable to understand why they can't have the feeling of full health despite doing everything "right."

DR. M'S GOALS FOR THE READER

The terms "leaky gut" and "leaky gut syndrome" are not synonymous. By end of this book, I hope that the reader will be able to understand the following:

- What is it that leaks?

- Where does it leak to?

- What causes the gut to leak?

- Are there tests available to check if your gut is leaky?

- What are the diseases linked to leaky gut?

- Can leaky gut affect organs beyond our intestines e.g. skin, brain, etc.?

What are the basic concepts underlying strengthening gut barrier and healing damaged barrier?

PRESENTATION OF A HOLISTIC APPROACH TO HEALING DISORDERED GUT

From my decades of experience as a physician, scientist, and educator, I have come to the conclusion that a reader cannot understand something that she skips over and does not read as happens in long paragraphs, especially in a health book.

The liberal use of short paragraphs and bulleted format makes this book easier to read and easier to understand and, as such, minimizes the potential for critical information being glossed over in the haystacks of larger paragraphs. I have, on purpose, made the chapters short; again to make the information easy to access and read. Some chapters are much shorter than others.

I have on occasion cited certain information or study more than once because of its relevance to the particular chapter and/or its significance because not everyone reads every word in any book. Such a repetition can also serve as a reminder for even the most avid reader.

Last but not the least, considering the significance of gut-brain connection, I have chosen to discuss the disorders associated with neurological dysfunction and chronic pain in distinct sections of their own.

BARRIOLOGY: THE NEW SCIENTIFIC FIELD FOCUSING ON GUT BARRIER

While the significance of gut barrier and importance of leaky gut was pooh-poohed as recently as a decade ago, more and more symposia at national scientific meetings of different specialties are now being devoted to discuss the significance of disordered gut and its milieu.

- Scientists are increasingly appreciating the critical significance of gut barrier in health and sickness.

- The term "Barriology" as a specialty has been proposed by Dr. Schoichiro Tsukita from the Osaka University in Osaka, Japan.

- Barriology involves the study of physiology of and diseased states involving intestinal barrier function of *tight junctions* between cells of the intestinal wall.

- Recent advances suggest that *tight junctions* are not just involved in fence and barrier function but also play a key role in day to day immune function of the gut, the body along with continued education of our body's immune system. This is a critical function since our gut is the body's largest immune organ.

WHAT HAS CHANGED OR NOT CHANGED IN RECENT TIMES?

Diseases are not solely determined by the genes but also the manifestation of genes based on their interaction with the environment. Infections, especially multidrug resistant infections, continue to be a problem especially in immune-compromised persons and at extremes of ages (e.g. infancy and elderly).

Overwhelming changes in our environment have occurred in recent decades:

- Global warming or climate changes.

- Migration from countryside to cities.

- Ever rising environmental pollution.

- Novel food engineering technologies that can change the amount or aggressiveness of allergenic or toxic substances humans are exposed to in everyday life.

- Changes in dietary habits with increasing emphasis on fast foods and preserved/canned foods etc.

The above changes are certain to affect our intestinal bacterial patterns in gut, air passages, as well as our skin. This, in turn, has the potential to alter our risk for diseases frequently linked to the gut like allergies, asthma, and atopic eczema.

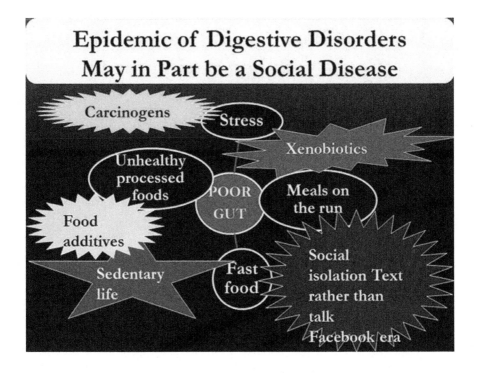

WHY DOES DISEASE NOT OCCUR IN EVERYONE UNDER SIMILAR CIRCUMSTANCES?

One might wonder why is everyone not sick, given the fact many people are exposed to similar dietary and environmental influences not just within families but also in similar neighborhoods. Genesis of disease is a complex phenomenon involving interaction of type and strength of attacking agent that can cause disease and the person's metabolic milieu and genes.

A mere presence of a gene does not increase or decrease the risk. A high risk gene when turned off may not pose any risk at all.

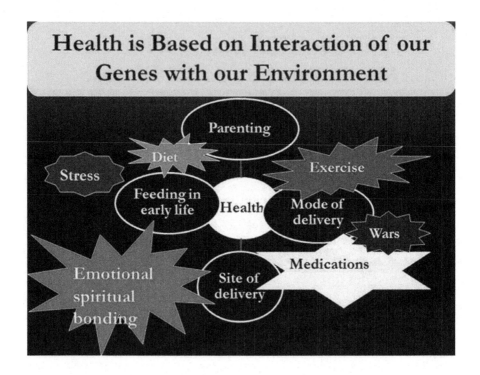

Potential scenarios

Healthy genes *Plus* low or no injury/toxin = No disease

Healthy genes *Plus* strong injury/toxin = Disease possible

Unhealthy genes *Plus* no injury/toxin = No disease

Unhealthy genes *Plus* strong injury/toxin = Disease

Unhealthy genes *Plus* low or weak injury/toxin = Disease possible

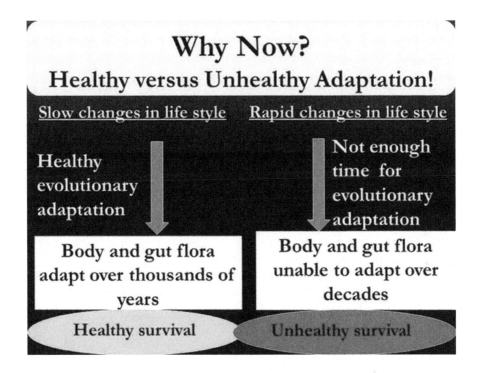

Diabetes type 1 is a prime example of diseases wherein a complex interaction of genetic and environmental factors determines the causation of the disease in an individual.

REFERENCES

1. Tsukita S, Yamazaki Y, Katsuno T et al. Tight junction-based epithelial microenvironment and cell proliferation. *Oncogene.* 2008 Nov24;27(55):6930-8.

2. Stankov K, Benc D, Draskovic D. Genetic and epigenetic factors in etiology of diabetes mellitus type 1. *Pediatrics.* 2013 Dec;132(6):1112-22.

CHAPTER 2

Healthy Gut

KEY POINTS

- Our digestive system is constantly performing digestive and protective functions throughout our lives.

- Gut is the largest immune organ in the body.

- Gut has a nervous system of its own.

If the matter is one that can be settled by observation, make the observation yourself. Aristotle could have avoided the mistake of thinking that women have fewer teeth than men, by the simple device of asking Mrs. Aristotle to keep her mouth open while he counted.

— *Bertrand Russell*

Our gut is a hard working organ which is in action 24/7, whether we are awake or asleep. Some of the well-known functions of the gut are as follows:

- Allows optimal digestive processing of consumed food and efficient absorption of nutrients.

- Ignores unneeded substances.

- Fights off potentially noxious substances.

- Eliminates luminal waste efficiently.

A healthy intestinal barrier is critical to not just intestinal health but to overall health throughout the body.

HEALTHY DYNAMIC BALANCE OF 5 FACTORS IS A PREREQUISITE FOR A HEALTHY GUT/BODY

While we all liken our human body to an extremely complex computer with a multitude of hardwiring and intricately connected software, the gut is frequently dismissed as just a simple organ to take care of the nutrition part. Such thinking about the role of the gut in our body is naïve to say the least.

In fact, many have lamented that it is the "forgotten organ" although this notion is being corrected as our knowledge grows. The gut has perhaps the most complex diversity of structure and function of all the organ systems in the human body. After all, it is not just responsible for nutrition.

Not only is the gut the largest organ per say, it is the largest immune organ, the largest hormone producing organ, and the largest organ exposed to trillions of bacteria all the time. With trillions of bacteria inside the gut, it makes the human body not just one living organism but rather a super-organism or our own discreet micro-universe!

Wait, there is more. The gut has a mind of its own, literally. Our gut's enteric nervous system has more cells in it than the peripheral nervous system in the rest of the body. It thinks and reacts on its own with some guidance from our big brain in the head.

A healthy gut is a must for overall health of the human body. Such a healthy state can only be maintained by an intricately balanced state comprising of the following factors:

- Digestion, absorption and assimilation.
- Intestinal barrier.
- Normal bacterial residents in the gut.
- Nervous system of the gut or enteric nervous system (ENS).
- Immune cells lining the gut or mucosal immune system.

Enteric nervous system (ENS), with some guidance from our big brain or central nervous system (CNS), controls the gastrointestinal functioning including digestion, absorption, intestinal movements, and secretions. It is crucial for our overall health.

THE GUT IS A DYNAMIC STAGE WITH ONGOING DIALOGUE OR CROSS-TALK AMONG ACTORS

The bacteria in the gut are not just sitting there for nothing or just waiting to attack the body. They are there to serve some very useful purposes. *Louis Pasteur* (1822-1895) once stated that life without microbes would be impossible.

The gut and its surrounding environment can be likened to a well-choreographed opera where a number of actors are singing and dancing in a well-organized fashion. This complex dancing does not stop the actors from talking between themselves on stage, something that does actually happen but we never hear!

Following are just some of the examples of intestinal actors involved in talking to each other and how this bidirectional messaging system has good or bad effects on the gut.

- Bacteria < —- > nerve cells of the intestinal nervous system altering motility and secretions

- Gut bacteria < ——— > intestinal wall and immune cells

- "Inter-kingdom" signaling among different types of bacteria causing sickness or healing

- Dysbiosis or abnormal unhealthy gut bacteria can alter motility further altering the gut bacteria towards the unhealthy gut à alters flora

Weakened intestinal integrity or leaky gut allows bacterial breakdown products, toxins, semi-digested allergenic dietary proteins and pro-inflammation signals direct access to nerve endings in the gut.

REFERENCES

1. Rosenstiel P. Stories of love and hate: innate immunity and host-microbe crosstalk in the intestine. *Curr Opin Gastroenterol.* 2013 Mar; 29(2):125-32.

2. Lipinski S, Rosenstiel P. Debug Your Bugs - How NLRs Shape Intestinal Host-Microbe Interactions. *Front Immunol.* 2013 Dec 27;4:479.

CHAPTER 3

Intestinal Barrier

KEY POINTS

- Intestinal barrier separates our body from gut lumen which contains trillions of bacteria, food, and toxins.

- The barrier, by necessity, is selectively porous. It has to allow nutritious substances to be absorbed while keeping the harmful substances at bay.

BARRAGE OF TOXIC INSULTS

We are constantly being subjected to a volley of chemical, physical, and biological insults not just from the outside environment but also from inside the gut. The body is protected from the intestinal attacks by the so-called intestinal barrier.

- The intestinal barrier is highly selective and semi-porous.

- A disjointed gut barrier exposes the gut (and, indirectly, the rest of the body) to trillions of micro-organisms, as well as potentially damaging foreign substances, undigested or semi-digested food components, and toxins.

- Bad substances come in direct contact with the intestinal nerve endings as well as gut immune system via a leaky barrier. This causes abnormal stimulation, leading to infection, unregulated inflammation, or neurogenic dysfunction at distant sites in the body.

The integrity of the gut barrier is affected by many internal factors including the gut bacteria, the food we eat, our daily lifestyle, and the stresses we encounter every day.

15

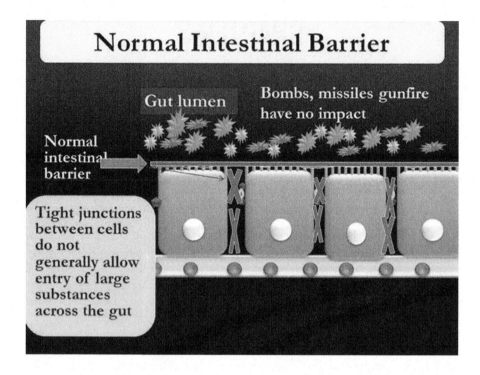

A SINGLE LAYER OF GUT CELLS SEPARATES BODY FROM POOP

The inside lumen of the gut actually is technically outside the body. It is an amazing feat of nature's creation that a single microscopic layer of cells separates our body from attack by trillions of bacteria as well as toxins in the gut and can still efficiently keep them apart. This microscopic layer of cells is an indispensable component of the intestinal barrier that performs critical bodily functions.

- Allows the body to communicate with the environment.
- Differentiates between friend and enemy.
- Healthy gut flora strengthen barrier.

- Interaction of the gut bacteria with the intestinal barrier results in a healthy immune system and creates a controlled state of inflammation to thwart attacks on the body by foreign materials/bacteria.

Leaky gut, altered gut bacteria, or dysfunctional biofilm can have profound consequences for education and subsequent regulation, function and control of the body's immune system.

> An abnormal immune activation can create uncontrolled inflammation in the gut that can spread throughout body.

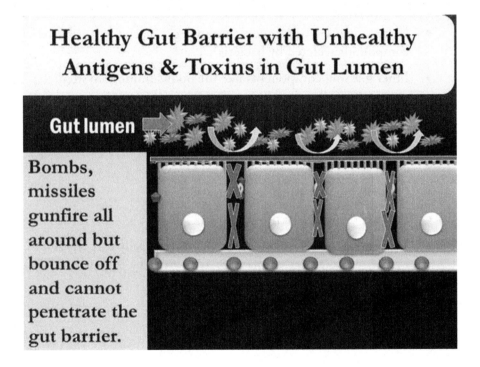

Healthy Gut Barrier with Unhealthy Antigens & Toxins in Gut Lumen

Gut lumen

Bombs, missiles gunfire all around but bounce off and cannot penetrate the gut barrier.

Composition of intestinal barrier

The intestinal barrier is complex in its structure and function. It is composed of several components that are in a dynamic state interacting with each other, with the rest of the human body, as well as with the intestinal milieu. The components of the barrier include:

- Biofilm.

- Digestive juices.

- Cell lining of the intestinal wall.

- Tight link-joints between the intestinal cells known as *tight junctions*.

- Outer mucus layer (mucin, normal gut bacteria, antibacterial compounds secreted by bacteria).

- Inner gut wall components like the body's immune system.

What is a Biofilm?

- Collectively unique ecological niche.

- Sticks to gut wall.

- Only 30 microns thick "pond scum".

- Protects the lining of the gut.

- Metabolizes undigested food remnants especially carbohydrates.

- May communicate with the body's immune system.

Inflammation is associated with a decrease in thickness of biofilm along with an increase in intestinal permeability or leakiness.

REFERENCES

1. Jeon MK, Klaus C, Kaemmerer E, Gassler N. Intestinal barrier: Molecular pathways and modifiers. *World J Gastrointest Pathophysiol.* 2013 Nov 15;4(4):94-99.

2. Camilleri M, Madsen K, Spiller R et al. Intestinal barrier function in health and gastrointestinal disease. *Neurogastroenterol Motil.* 2012 Jun;24(6):503-12.

3. Scaldaferri F, Pizzoferrato M, Gerardi V et al. The gut barrier: new acquisitions and therapeutic approaches. *J Clin Gastroenterol.* 2012 Oct;46 Suppl:S12-7.

CHAPTER 4

The Gut: Is it Leaky or Not Leaky?

KEY POINTS

- Gut barrier is semi-permeable and made up of pores of small and large size.

- Substances may go across the gut wall through the cells or in-between the cells.

- The lining between the cells is linked by complex and dynamic structures known as *tight junctions*.

Although this may seem a paradox, all exact science is dominated by the idea of approximation. When a man tells you that he knows the exact truth about anything, you are safe in inferring that he is an inexact man. Every careful measurement in science is always given with the probable error ... every observer admits that he is likely wrong and knows about how much wrong he is likely to be.

— *Bertrand Russell*

The gut by definition is porous or leaky. After all, it has to be able to absorb substances needed for the body.

PASSAGE OF SUBSTANCES
ACROSS THE GUT WALL

Two pathways are involved

- Trans-cellular (i.e. transport through the cells of the intestine).

- Para-cellular (i.e. transport between the adjacent cells of the gut wall).

Pores in the gut

The gut has pores of various sizes. While smaller compounds can be absorbed through smaller pores, larger substances are limited by having to use larger pores that are less accessible and less in number.

When we use the term leaky gut, we imply that the gut barrier allows passage across the gut of substances larger than a certain size (molecular weight of 150 Da) and many of these can be toxic to our system. These include semi-digested foods components.

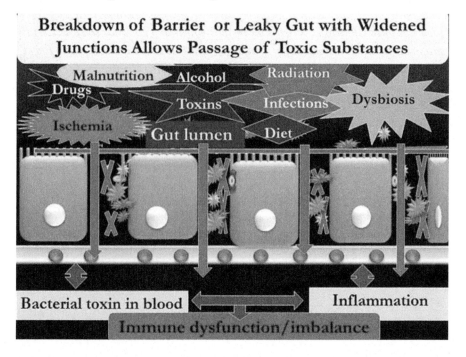

Our ability to test for leaky gut is limited by the fact that we are only able to assess passage of water-soluble compounds but not the fat soluble substances! Even the available tests do not appear to be very sensitive and show different results based on the probe used.

The intestinal barrier is very complex. It separates the body from the fecal matter full of potentially harmful bacteria and other harmful substances in the gut. While well-maintained during the course of evolution of millions of years, the barrier is not impervious.

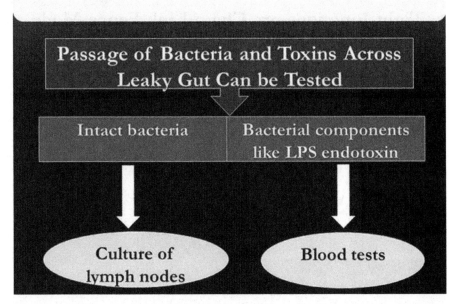

TIGHT JUNCTIONS

GUT WALL IS LIKE CHAIN FENCE

Think of the cell lining of the gut wall as a chain link fence. *Tight junctions* are links between the cells of the intestinal lining and help them stay connected. However, *tight junctions* are not like barriers made of concrete and steel.

After all, a very important function of the digestive system is to digest and absorb the nutrients that we consume. The critical function of absorption can only be successful if the nutrients required for our sustenance can cross the gut barrier.

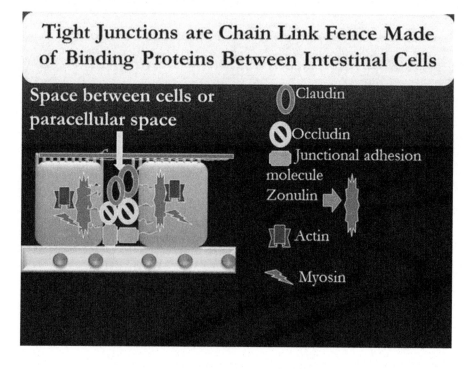

TIGHT JUNCTIONS ARE PICKY

The selectivity of tight junctions is based on its unique structural and functional properties. These include the following:

- Comprised of dynamic structures including proteins.

- Selective leakiness based on size and electrical charge on the substances trying to cross the pores of the barrier.

- Rapid and coordinated responses.

- Important for movement of fluid and solutes.

- Alter permeability or leakiness depending upon environment.

- *Zonulin* component of tight junctions is involved in controlling as gatekeeper and has been implicated in many pathological disorders.

  o Induces rearrangement of cytoskeleton

  o Disrupts complex integrity

  o Increases permeability or leakiness

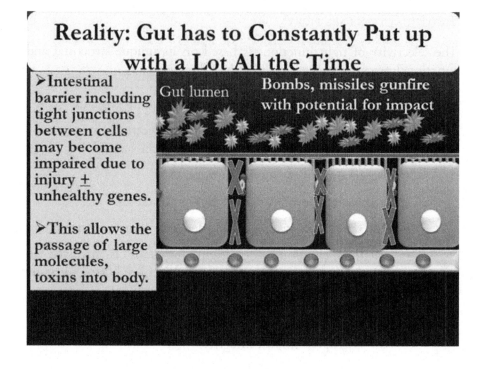

Reality: Gut has to Constantly Put up with a Lot All the Time

➢Intestinal barrier including tight junctions between cells may become impaired due to injury ± unhealthy genes.

➢This allows the passage of large molecules, toxins into body.

Gut lumen

Bombs, missiles gunfire with potential for impact

REFERENCES

1. Peterson LW, Artis D. Intestinal epithelial cells: regulators of barrier function and immune homeostasis. *Nat Rev Immunol.* 2014 Mar;14(3):141-53.

2. Fasano A. Intestinal permeability and its regulation by zonulin: diagnostic and therapeutic implications. *Clin Gastroenterol Hepatol.* 2012 Oct;10(10):1096-100.

CHAPTER 5

Factors Affecting Gut Leakiness

KEY POINTS

- Numerous human, dietary, intestinal and lifestyle factors have an impact on intestinal barrier.

- Intestinal bacteria play a critical role in maintaining a healthy intestinal barrier.

- Gut depends on normal gut bacteria for barrier integrity.

We are ... led to a somewhat vague distinction between what we may call "hard" data and "soft" data. This distinction is a matter of degree, and must not be pressed; but if not taken too seriously it may help to make the situation clear.

— Bertrand Russell

A delicate equilibrium between the intestinal bacteria and immune cells of the gut must exist in order to maintain reliability of healthy function of the intestine. Multiple interactions are involved in immune cells tolerating normal bacterial inhabitants and food proteins, while attacking toxins and disease-producing bacteria.

- The intestinal cells and its resident immune cells do not simply tolerate normal bacterial inhabitants – they depend on them.

- Some passage of bacteria across the gut wall occurs all the time for "checking up." This allows the body to sample intestinal bacteria and proteins so the gut can mount a controlled immune reaction to foreign proteins and bad bacteria.

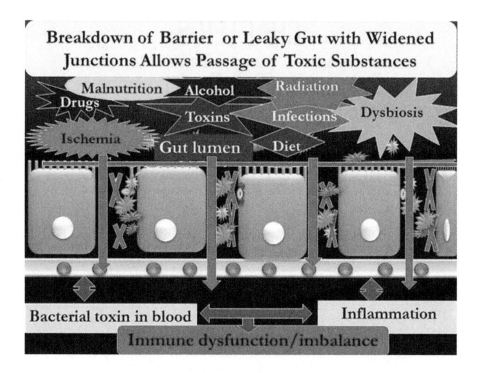

EFFECT OF CHANGES IN INTESTINAL BACTERIA

Alterations of gut bacteria can have profound implications across the entire body. The complex interactions between harmful intestinal bacteria and the cells of the intestinal wall can disrupt the intestinal barrier, alter fluid and electrolyte absorption pathways, and provoke an inflammation that can spread throughout body.

Functional abnormalities in *tight junctions* can be seen in inflammation and autoimmune diseases, including inflammatory bowel disease, type I diabetes, and celiac disease.

Selectively getting rid of intestinal bacteria reduces respiratory infections in critically ill patients. Probiotics can help reduce the prevalence of disease-producing bacteria in the gut and help reduce infections after surgical operations. The mechanisms include boosting immunity and strengthening the gut barrier.

HUMAN FACTORS

Age: Intestinal leakiness is higher at infancy and old age. The leakiness is especially high in premature babies.

Pregnancy: High stress is a risk factor for spontaneous abortion. Stress increases intestinal leakiness, allowing passage of partially-digested food, bacteria, and toxins into the body. This, in turn, provokes abnormal activation of the immune system producing inflammation. This affects a pregnant woman's acclimatization and adjustment to pregnancy, and the baby in the womb is then perceived as foreign. Strengthening the intestinal barrier and restoration of immune tolerance by use of probiotics may offer a new therapeutic target in such cases.

Exercise: Heat stress during exercise causes a decrease in blood flow to the gut since blood goes preferentially to exercising muscles. This disrupts the intestinal barrier. Dr. Smetanka and colleagues from the University of Iowa studied marathon runners who took ibuprofen prior to and during running. These runners developed intestinal leakiness, demonstrated by increased lactulose in the blood and in urine. Half of the runners also developed symptoms of a GI infection.

ENVIRONMENTAL FACTORS

Farm environment: Contact with farm animals contributes to the protective *"farm effect"* and strengthens the gut barrier. A pregnant woman's exposure to animal sheds during pregnancy offers a protective benefit for the baby. The umbilical cord in such cases has higher levels of antibodies, as well as other protective interferon chemicals.

DIETARY FACTORS

Diet: The diet affects *tight junctions* as well as immune functions.

- The intestinal barrier is impaired in patients with kidney failure, but it can be restored to normal when patients eat a low-protein diet.

- Consumption of formula diet with pre-digested proteins improves Crohn's disease symptoms.

- Potato skins worsen intestinal permeability and aggravate inflammatory bowel disease in animals. Avoid a high-potato diet, especially fried potatoes.

- Excessive dietary fat causes an increase in intestinal leakiness. Genetic obesity does not play a role in risk due to fat. While certain fats dilate the tight junctions, omega-3 fatty acids actually strengthen the barrier via their anti-inflammation action. Butyrate, a short chain fatty acid, enhances the barrier function.

- Rapid fermentation of a high FODMAPs diet produces excess acids, gases (hydrogen, carbon dioxide, methane, and hydrogen sulfide), and surfactants that reduce surface tension. These factors mess up the intestinal barrier. FODMAPs have been implicated in the rising tide of a variety of conditions like Crohn's disease, celiac disease, IBS, chronic fatigue syndrome, and autism.

- Milk fat has adverse effects in animal colitis, whereas fermented milk is beneficial. Infants consuming only formula show 2.8 times more intestinal leakiness compared to those receiving some human milk.

- Consumption of unprocessed cow's milk protects against disruption of intestinal barrier. This protection can also be seen in non-farm kids ingesting unpasteurized cow's milk. (I am not advocating drinking unpasteurized milk.)

- Hot spices like black and red pepper have a digestive stimulant action and heal digestive disorders. Inflammation is a pivotal component of numerous diverse diseases, such as atherosclerosis and cancer. Studies suggest possible strengthening of the intestinal barrier by hot peppers. However, the effects in damaged epithelium may be quite the opposite.

GUT LEAKINESS AND FOOD PROCESSING

One of biggest components of foreign material in our gut is food itself. It should not then be a surprise that not just the type of food itself but also the condition of the food can affect the gut barrier.

The role of *advanced glycation end products* (AGEs) and glycated lipids is important.

- AGEs can be absorbed into the body if the gut is leaky.

- Amount type of AGEs depends on type of cooking.

- AGEs have been implicated in allergy and metabolic syndrome.

- Glycation of food allergens increases their potential to cause immune reaction in the body.

  o Strongly roasting peanuts increases its allergenicity.

  o Broiling and frying is worse than roasting.

  o Boiling is best.

WATER AND FLUID INTAKE

Avoid carbonated beverages. Drink at least 8 glasses of water per day unless restricted by a physician. While it is true that the amount of water consumed by healthy subjects does not have a significant impact, such comparative studies have not been performed in diseased states and in those with leaky gut.

- Low-mineral water improves intestinal leakiness in patients with skin eczema.

- Dehydration increases intestinal leakiness. The increase in permeability is subdued in subjects receiving fluids during exercise.

- Maintain adequate hydration, even during a short fast. Prolonged fasting combined with stress leads to intestinal damage as well as the passage of partially-digested dietary proteins, bacteria, and toxins from the gut into the body across a leaky gut. Fasting for a couple of days with adequate hydration should not be a problem in adequately nourished persons.

FOOD COMPONENTS AFFECTING TIGHT JUNCTIONS IN THE GUT WALL

Factors disrupting tight junctions

- Food surfactants like sucrose monoester fatty acid, a food grade surfactant.
- Sodium caprate, a medium chain lipid.

Factors strengthening tight junctions

- Glutamine
- Butyrate
- Turmeric
- Zinc
- Vitamin D

POTENTIAL TOXINS THAT WE CONSUME

GLIADIN/GLUTEN

Gluten is a well-known toxin from grains like wheat, rye and barley. It is a big problem in patients with celiac disease. Gliadin is a semi-digested breakdown product of dietary gluten. Celiac disease happens as a result of a failure of *tight junctions* causing increased leakiness and absorption of the food protein gliadin.

However, one does not have to have celiac disease to have problems due to gluten. For years, many patients with irritable bowel syndrome had been reporting improvement of their symptoms upon exclusion of gluten from their diet.

Such reports were dismissed by physicians (including myself) for a long time despite evidence from initial studies done decades ago.

Fortunately, even more science has finally caught up with public perception. Recent studies have clearly substantiated patients' claims of improvement of IBS symptoms upon exclusion of gluten from diet.

The condition has been labeled as "non-celiac gluten sensitivity or intolerance." Gliadin has also been implicated in the pathogenesis of a variety of other autoimmune disorders.

Food surfactants

Food-grade surfactants are common additives in foods that we buy from the grocery store. These surfactants cause separation of the *tight junctions* and allow increased passage of harmful protein breakdown products across the gut wall into the body.

Alcohol

Alcohol intake, both acute and chronic, disrupts intestinal barrier via multiple actions, including inflammation, oxidative stress, and histamines. Alcoholic subjects have five times higher levels of intestinal bacterial toxin in their blood than healthy controls. The alcohol-induced intestinal permeability promotes abnormal passage of bacterial toxin across the gut wall and into the blood stream, causing damage to distant organs. This is thought to be a big factor in causing alcoholic liver disease. Acute consumption of alcohol also causes gastrointestinal ulcers.

According to Dr. Keshavarzian and colleagues from the Rush University Medical Center, Chicago and as published in the *Journal of Hepatology* in 2009:

- Chronic alcoholism makes the gut become leaky as determined by the lactulose-mannitol absorption test.

- There is an increased level of intestinal bacterial toxin in the blood indicating that the toxin is able to pass across the leaky gut into the body of chronic alcoholics.

- There is increased evidence of oxidative stress indicating the body's antioxidant defensives are coming up short.

- The above changes occur concurrently with increasing fat in the liver leading to fatty liver.

A chemical may have a toxic effect in one person and benefits in another depending on the make-up of genes and the quantity of the toxin. Above notwithstanding, moderate drinking, especially red wine, has been associated with positive health outcomes. Data on the effect of smoking on the intestinal barrier is mixed.

THERAPEUTIC STATES

Surgery: In addition to the effects of fasting, handling of the gut during surgery itself affects the intestinal barrier. For example, gallbladder surgery: when using tiny incisions during laparoscopic cholecystectomy, causes much less of an increase in intestinal permeability and increase in blood levels of bacterial endotoxin, as compared to the open surgical approach using one big incision.

Iron: Taking iron pills increases intestinal leakiness. This could be one of the mechanisms explaining the negative effects of medicinal iron supplementation on health.

Nonsteroidal anti-inflammatory drugs (NSAIDs): NSAIDs cause abnormalities of the intestinal barrier. NSAIDs reduce energy production by the cells, thus impairing the *tight junctions*. Chronic use of NSAIDs causes ulcers and bleeding, along with precipitating relapses in patients with inflammatory bowel disease.

Mental state and stress: The role of psychological stress and anxiety in health and sickness is being increasingly recognized. Stress alters the fluid and electrolyte balance, mucus secretion, along with structural and functional changes of gut barrier making the gut leaky. Alterations in intestinal barrier function can be demonstrated in experimental animal models of acute as well as chronic stress.

- Rats separated from their mothers show increased sensitivity to pain and increased bowel movements, suggesting disrupted intestinal barrier.

- Stress worsens colitis in animal models of inflammatory bowel disease. Stress and anxiety are involved in the causation and worsening of functional bowel disorders like IBS. Stressed patients are more likely to suffer relapses of functional and inflammatory disorders.

Dr. Catassi and colleagues from the Università Politecnica delle Marche in Italy characterize non-celiac gluten sensitivity as the new frontier of gluten-related disorders. Gluten sensitivity may be involved in organs far removed from the gut itself. Drs. Genuis and Lobo (2014) from the University of Alberta in Edmonton, Canada argue that gluten sensitivity may present as neuropsychiatric disorders like autism, schizophrenia, and ataxia.

MISCELLANEOUS FACTORS AFFECTING GUT PERMEABILITY OR LEAKINESS

NORMAL FACTORS IN A HEALTHY PERSON

- Programmed cell death
- Inflammation
- Intestinal bacteria

- Biochemicals involved in nerve signaling and inflammation
- Immune cells

ABNORMAL FACTORS

- Intestinal obstruction
- Poor or lack of blood supply to the gut
- Jaundice
- Inflammatory bowel disease
- Cancer
- Trauma, including surgery
- Infections
- Slow gut
- Small intestinal bacterial overgrowth

The intestinal barrier is a highly complex structure that allows for selective permeability. Intestinal contents including diet, drugs, and intestinal bacteria interact with the gut barrier. Indirectly, they interact and communicate with the body's immune cells and nerve cells. These processes play a critical role in health and sickness. Simple things, like being fed on breast milk or formula milk during infancy, may have long-term consequences.

REFERENCES

1. Man AL, Gicheva N, Nicoletti C. The impact of ageing on the intestinal epithelial barrier and immune system. *Cell Immunol.* 2014 Apr 12;289(1-2):112-118.

2. Price D, Ackland L, Suphioglu C. Nuts 'n' guts: transport of food

allergens across the intestinal epithelium. *Asia Pac Allergy.* 2013 Oct;3(4):257-65.

3. Biesiekierski JR, Newnham ED, Irving PM et al. Gluten causes gastrointestinal symptoms in subjects without celiac disease: a double-blind randomized placebo-controlled trial. *Am J Gastroenterol.* 2011 Mar;106(3):508-14.

4. Keshavarzian A, Farhadi A, Forsyth CB et al. Evidence that chronic alcohol exposure promotes intestinal oxidative stress, intestinal hyperpermeability and endotoxemia prior to development of alcoholic steatohepatitis in rats. *J Hepatol.* 2009 Mar;50(3):538-47.

5. Chen P, Schnabl B. Host-Microbiome Interactions in Alcoholic Liver Disease. *Gut Liver.* 2014 May;8(3):237-241.

6. DA Silva S, Robbe-Masselot C, Ait-Belgnaoui A et al. Stress disrupts intestinal mucus barrier in rats via mucin O-glycosylation shift: prevention by a probiotic treatment. *Am J Physiol Gastrointest Liver Physiol.* 2014 Jun 26.

7. Kerr CA, Grice DM, Tran CD et al. Early life events influence whole-of-life metabolic health via gut microflora and gut permeability. *Crit Rev Microbiol.* 2014 Mar 19.

CHAPTER 6

Leaky Gut Barrier

KEY POINTS

- Inflammation and leaky gut worsen each other.
- Leaky gut weakens the immune system, increasing the risk for allergic, inflammatory, and autoimmune diseases.

Disruption of healthy patterns of intestinal bacteria in early life results in a poorly educated and trained immune system of not just the gut, but the entire body. This has potential to act like an uncontrolled brat later on in life with resultant chronic illnesses.

The structural and functional integrity of dynamic *tight junctions* (TJs) is indispensable for maintaining a healthy balance of selective intestinal penetrability. Inflammation disrupts these *tight junctions*, increasing intestinal permeability and creating a so-called "leaky gut." This allows toxins and foreign proteins to cross the intestinal barrier and interact with our internal tissues.

INFLAMMATION AND LEAKY BARRIER ARE INTER-LINKED

Inflammation and leaky barrier worsen each other. A variety of mechanisms are involved in inflammation and leaky gut exacerbating each other and the resultant disease manifestations. The following examples illustrate this point:

INFLAMMATORY BOWEL DISEASE

The inciting substance is the gut bacteria leading to increased inflammation as seen by an increase in tumor necrosis factor (TNF). Remission can be attained by using drugs that block tumor necrosis factor or anti-TNF drugs. These drugs also decrease intestinal permeability reducing gut leakiness.

GRAFT VERSUS HOST DISEASE

The inciting antigen is from a person's own body stimulating inflammation and TNF. Disease can be controlled by anti-TNF drugs.

CELIAC SPRUE

The foreign antigen is the gluten from the diet causing inflammation. Anti-TNF drugs suppress the disease. Celiac sprue is classic leaky gut and is associated with a variety of autoimmune diseases.

EFFECTS OF LEAKY GUT

Intestinal barrier is a highly selective barrier between the gut lumen full of crap and gut immune cells; yet, it is a porous wall.

- Defective digestion and absorption of nutrients.

- Weakened immune system of the gut.

- Large, undigested or semi-digested proteins from food, bacteria, or toxins can enter body, perceived as foreigners causing the body to set off an immune reaction to fight these invaders. This, in turn, increases the potential to set off diseases characterized by unregulated inflammation like allergic and autoimmune diseases.

- Bacteria communicate with the brain via direct access to the nerve endings in the gut.

HEALTHY GUT

Intestinal sensing cells are in contact with bacteria in intestinal lumen on one side and the nerve endings in the gut wall on the other. These cells produce signaling chemicals like serotonin (5HT) which *convey* bidirectional signals to and from the gut and the brain.

Over 90% of the body's 5HT is contained in the gut. Of note, commonly used antidepressant medications that act via 5HT are used not just for the brain but also for intestinal disorders like irritable bowel syndrome.

UNHEALTHY GUT

Increased leakiness of the gut allows bacterial chemical signals direct access to intestinal nerve endings without the editorial influence of intestinal sensing cells and as such are able to communicate directly with our brain. Such unregulated signals-communications with the brain have the potential for neurobehavioral, psychiatric and chronic pain syndromes.

IS LEAKY GUT OR INCREASED INTESTINAL PERMEABILITY A DISEASE?

- Not a specific disease in itself but a disordered process.
- Allows toxins and antigens access to body.
- Increased inflammatory, metabolic stress.
- Disease manifestations depending on multiple factors including a person's genes.
- Proposed as precursor to autoimmune diseases.

POTENTIAL CONSEQUENCES OF LEAKY GUT IN EARLY LIFE

Disruption of healthy patterns and relationships of intestinal bacteria in early life (e.g. infections, antibiotic use) can damage the gut's learning ability on how to discriminate and make distinction between normal bacterial inhabitants and the unhealthy, disease-producing bacteria.

The body's immune system goes into an attack mode, and this can trigger uncontrolled inflammation, setting the stage for further leakiness in a vicious cycle. This creates a perfect environment for the person to suffer from chronic allergic and autoimmune diseases.

REFERENCES

1. Scalera A, Di Minno MN, Tarantino G. What does irritable bowel syndrome share with non-alcoholic fatty liver disease? *World J Gastroenterol.* 2013 Sep 7;19(33):5402-20.

2. Peterson LW, Artis D. Intestinal epithelial cells: regulators of barrier function and immune homeostasis. *Nat Rev Immunol.* 2014 Mar;14(3):141-53.

3. Goto Y, Ivanov II. Intestinal epithelial cells as mediators of the commensal-host immune crosstalk. *Immunol Cell Biol.* 2013 Mar;91(3):204-14.

CHAPTER 7

How Does Leaky Gut Cause its Effects

KEY POINTS

- Leaky gut is not a theoretical phenomenon.
- Oxidative burst is essential for body defenses when it occurs in a controlled fashion.
- Multiple chemical sensitivity syndrome can occur.

William James used to preach the "will to believe." For my part, I should wish to preach the "will to doubt." … What is wanted is not the will to believe, but the wish to find out, which is the exact opposite.
— Bertrand Russell

WHAT HAPPENS IN LEAKY GUT

TIGHT JUNCTIONS OPEN

- Translocation of bacteria occurs.
- Bacteria, toxins, semi-digested dietary proteins, and allergenic substances or antigens have direct access to the body by entering into the systemic blood circulation.
    - Do not have to go through the lymph nodes and portal vein.
    - Potentially toxic substances evade body's immune defenses.

CHAIN REACTION OF TRANSLOCATION

The opening of leaky channels allows bacteria to engage immune white blood cells at the surface of the gut. Bacteria can then move across the gut and into the blood stream to reach the entire body. This bypasses the normal passage through the liver via the portal vein, thus circumvents the body's detoxification methods. This bacterial translocation can cause inflammation at distant sites.

- Bacteria start fighting with the body's defensive white blood cells at the surface of the gut. This releases inflammation promoting compounds as well as activated white blood cells into the body.

- The inflammatory processes and molecules can be carried to distant sites resulting in stimulation of immune system at distant organs of the body.

- Because of leaky gut, there is a greater release of inflammatory chemicals and activated white blood cells without corresponding suppressive anti-inflammatory signals to tone down the inflammation.

- Abnormal proteins, bacteria, and toxins are carried to distant organs like the lungs etc.

- Activation of the immune system at the distant sites (lungs, liver, kidney, etc.) occurs.

OUTBURST OF REACTIVE OXYGEN SPECIES

The activated white blood cells cause a massive outburst of reactive oxygen species as part of the fighting mechanisms. This increases inflammation and oxidative stress in different organs.

The oxidative burst, when not adequately confronted by the body's antioxidant mechanisms, results in further weakening of the gut barrier and disease in various organs may occur.

> Unchallenged inflammation is analogous to bombs, missiles, and grenades which are hurled from a defensive site (e.g. the gut) to cause explosions at distant sites (lungs, liver, heart, kidney, and brain.)

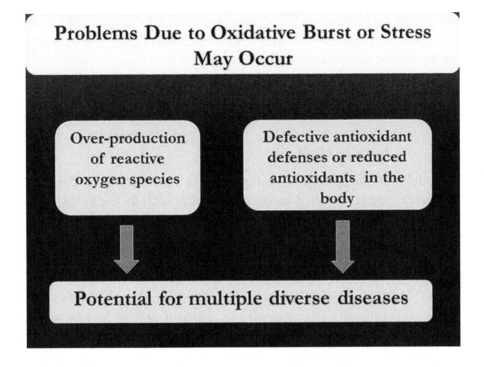

OXIDATIVE BURST IN AN ATTACK MODE

Oxidative burst is a rapid production of various toxic and chemically active derivatives known as reactive oxygen species (ROS) especially by immune cells.

- Common ROS generated include:
  - Superoxide
  - Hydrogen peroxide
- Occurs in response to engagement with foreign materials such as invading bacteria etc.
- The above results in a spike in metabolic reactions in the cells.

In a healthy state, the oxidative burst and the resultant chemicals attack the foreign substances to destroy them. However, this action has to occur in a controlled fashion with antioxidant defenses calming the oxidative outburst as its need subsides.

The mismatch between excess of ROS and inadequate defenses increases the potential for multiple diverse diseases.

OXIDATIVE BURST IN LEAKY GUT

Harmful immune processes and metabolic reactions initiated at the leaky gut barrier are transported to the distant sites such as the lungs, liver, heart, and kidney via circulation.

- More like dangerous explosives in the form of bombs, missiles, and grenades thrown from a distant battle ship during the war.

- The signals that calm the oxidative burst and its resultant inflammatory processes may be deficient or may be blocked in some people due to their genes and other factors.

- Damage locally and/or at distant organs is explosive and can become sustained.

The resulting damage has been labeled by some as *"leaky gut or leaky membrane syndrome."*

OXIDATIVE BURST CAN EVEN BE LIFE-THREATENING

An oxidative burst does not necessarily affect just one or two organs. Depending on the circumstances, it may cause a life-threatening multi-organ failure.

ACTION

- Severe pro-inflammatory reaction

  Plus

- Inadequate anti-oxidant defenses or oxidative stress

RESULT = Multi-organ-failure

Multiple sensitivity syndrome may occur.

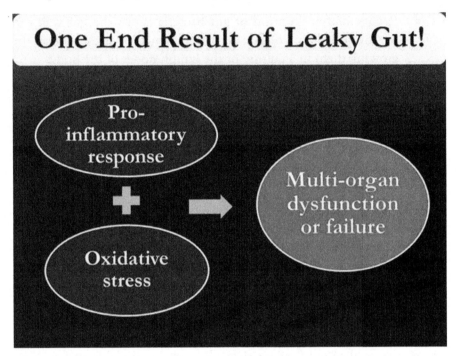

Absorbed toxins overwhelm the body's detox mechanisms making a person vulnerable to even minute amounts of chemicals i.e. multiple chemical sensitivity syndrome (fragrances, air fresheners, etc.).

BIOLOGICAL EVIDENCE OF LEAKY GUT

- Leaky gut is not just a theoretical phenomenon. Intestinal hyperpermeability is a well-established fact associated with many diseases. While the association of leaky gut with many diseases has been established, it is controversial if there is a cause-effect relationship. Not everyone agrees on the model of "leaky gut syndrome" as a cause of diseases.

- Passage or translocation of gut bacteria across the gut wall can be confirmed by confirming the presence of such bacteria by growing them in a culture of the lymph nodes of the body.

- Tests can confirm the presence of bacterial products/toxin in the blood, e.g. lipopolysaccharide (LPS) toxin.

- Blood tests can document the presence of antibodies against the intestinal bacterial toxin supporting the concept that passage of bacteria and toxins results in stimulating an immune reaction in the body.

LEAKY GUT AND MALABSORPTION CAN CO-EXIST

The concept of co-existence of leaky gut and poor absorption of nutrients is counter-intuitive. However, these two phenomena may co-exist. For example, decreased surface area of the gut wall seen in celiac with decreased absorption should theoretically decrease leakiness while the opposite is true. Permeability defect or leaky processes can best be explained as a disorder of the cells lining the gut wall and not simply loss of surface area. Absorption of digested food particles depends on available surface area; damaged microvilli of the gut wall are reduced in a variety of diseases like:

- Crohn's disease
- Celiac disease
- Radiation enteritis
- Gastrointestinal infections
- Medications like aspirin/NSAIDs

REFERENCES

1. Al-Gubory KH. Environmental pollutants and lifestyle factors induce oxidative stress and poor prenatal development. *Reprod Biomed Online*. 2014 Jul;29(1):17-31.

2. Rossignol DA, Frye RE. Evidence linking oxidative stress, mitochondrial dysfunction, and inflammation in the brain of individuals with autism. *Front Physiol*. 2014 Apr 22;5:150.3(14)00132-1.

3. Wright C, Milne S, Leeson H. Sperm DNA damage caused by oxidative stress: modifiable clinical, lifestyle and nutritional factors in male infertility. *Reprod Biomed Online*. 2014 Mar 4. pii: S1472-6483(14)00118-7.

4. De Luca C, Raskovic D, Pacifico V et al. The search for reliable biomarkers of disease in multiple chemical sensitivity and other environmental intolerances. *Int J Environ Res Public Health*. 2011 Jul;8(7):2770-97.

5. Genuis SJ. Sensitivity-related illness: the escalating pandemic of allergy, food intolerance and chemical sensitivity. *Sci Total Environ*. 2010 Nov 15;408(24):6047-61.

SECTION II

Diseases Associated with Leaky Gut

CHAPTER 8

Leaky Gut Syndrome

KEY POINTS

- While the evidence of a cause-effect relationship is evolving, clinical and experimental data suggests that leaky gut may be involved in causing and perpetuating many GI and non-GI diseases.

- Apparently, different diseases occur when the interaction of leaky barrier, abnormal gut bacteria, and abnormal immune reactions in genetically-vulnerable patients creates a "perfect storm" critical to the disease.

- Leaky gut may just be one part of the overall disease-causing mechanisms. Other external factors, including abnormal bacterial patterns, are involved.

The most savage controversies are those about matters as to which there is no good evidence either way.
— Bertrand Russell

WHAT CAME FIRST:
LEAKY GUT OR THE DISEASE

"Leaky gut syndrome" has been implicated in the causation and sustenance of a wide variety of diseases affecting different organ systems. Opinions differ on the basis of which came first, the chicken or the egg.

Although abnormal intestinal barrier function or leaky gut could just be a result of a disease, mounting evidence points to its involvement in *causing* and then sustaining the disease in a vicious cycle. The lines of evidence supporting this concept include, but are not limited to, the following:

- The presence of leaky gut prior to the onset of the disease itself.
- The presence of leaky gut in healthy relatives but not in healthy control subjects.

A disrupted barrier allows for bacteria and toxins to enter the body which provokes inflammation and oxidative reaction. A torrent of reactions ensues, depending upon the person's genes and environmental factors.

Even in cases where the leaky gut may not be the initial causative factor, once the disease sets in, leaky gut may occur as an effect. A vicious cycle may then occur with the leaky gut worsening the disease which in turn further loosens up the intestinal barrier.

UNHEALTHY GENE FOR LEAKY GUT DOES NOT EQUAL DISEASE

GENES MAY BE SILENT, OVER- OR UNDERACTIVE

Based on how the gene manifests (stays silent, becomes overactive, or is defective), different insults like inflammation, oxidative stress, and intestinal bacteria (does not always have to be abnormal bacteria) can lead to *leaky gut* and diverse disease manifestations or syndromes.

A variety of scenarios may occur in an assortment of combinations and permutations. There may be bacteria crossing the gut into the body or there may just be a passage of bacterial toxin or other toxins across the leaky gut into the body.

These foreign substances, if perceived as harmful, then cause an inflammatory reaction in the body as manifested by activated white blood cells and the production of inflammatory molecules. There is also an increase in stress hormones which, in turn, affect the immune, hormonal, as well as central and peripheral nervous systems.

> Healthy gut—> Infections, antibiotics, toxins, inflammation —>
> Leaky gut

REFERENCES

1. Odenwald MA, Turner JR. Intestinal permeability defects: is it time to treat? *Clin Gastroenterol Hepatol.* 2013 Sep;11(9):1075-83.

2. Lindros KO, Järveläinen HA. Chronic systemic endotoxin exposure: an animal model in experimental hepatic encephalopathy. *Metab Brain Dis.* 2005 Dec;20(4):393-8.

3. Anders HJ, Andersen K, Stecher B. The intestinal microbiota, a leaky gut, and abnormal immunity in kidney disease. *Kidney Int. 2013 Jun;83(6):1010-6.*

CHAPTER 9

Autoimmune Diseases of Various Kinds May Occur

KEY POINTS

- Prevalence of autoimmune disorders has been rising in recent decades.

- Infections, drugs, and toxins are common triggers of autoimmune disease.

- Leaky gut has been implicated in pathogenesis of many autoimmune diseases. Both the leaky gut and genetic predisposition must be present for the disease to occur.

- Screening for leaky gut has been advocated for people at high risk for autoimmune disease.

30-50 million Americans suffer from a variety of autoimmune diseases. Although much remains to be understood, common triggers of autoimmune diseases include:

- Bacteria

- Viruses

- Drugs

- Toxins

FEATURES OF AUTOIMMUNE DISEASE

Autoimmune diseases can be identified by circumstantial evidence, usually by one or more of the following features:

- Presence of auto-antibodies.

- Frequent co-occurrence with other autoimmune diseases likely due to similar genes.

- Female predisposition.

- Good response to immune-suppressive treatment.

ROLE OF TESTING FOR LEAKY GUT

Drs. Mishra and Makharia from the AIIMS in New Delhi, India have suggested the use of permeability testing to check for an increase in risk for certain autoimmune diseases. Success of this strategy bearing fruit was reported by Drs. Irvine and Marshall from the *McMaster University in Ontario, Canada*. A child found to have leaky gut during screening of family members of patients with Crohn's disease demonstrated onset of Crohn's disease 8 years later.

REFERENCES

1. Campbell AW. Autoimmunity and the gut. *Autoimmune Dis.* 2014;2014:152428.

2. Berer K, Krishnamoorthy G. Microbial view of central nervous system autoimmunity. *FEBS Lett.* 2014 Apr 18. pii: S0014-5793(14)00293-2.

3. Irvine EJ, Marshall JK. Increased intestinal permeability precedes the onset of Crohn's disease in a subject with familial risk. *Gastroenterology.* 2000 Dec;119(6):1740-4.

4. Shamir R, Shehadeh N. Insulin in human milk and the use of hormones in infant formulas. *Nestle Nutr Inst Workshop Ser.* 2013;77:57-64.

5. Mishra A, Makharia GK. Techniques of functional and motility test: how to perform and interpret intestinal permeability. *J Neurogastroenterol Motil.* 2012 Oct;18(4):443-7.

CHAPTER 10

Select Listing of Diseases Linked to Leaky Gut

KEY POINTS

- Leaky gut is associated with a wide variety of disorders involving diverse organ systems of the body.

- Many of these diseases tend to co-occur in the same individual.

INTERPRETING TESTS FOR LEAKY GUT

This book cites numerous studies documenting abnormalities on tests for intestinal permeability. Consider those tests in proper context. Bear in mind that most available tests for leaky gut are rudimentary.

None of the available tests can investigate all the possible pathways whereby noxious substances can cross between the adjacent cells and/or directly through the cells of the gut barrier. Available tests do not also test for passage of fat soluble substances.

GI DISEASES

- Celiac disease
- Crohn's disease
- Ulcerative colitis
- Irritable bowel syndrome
- Collagenous colitis
- Gastrointestinal infections
- NSAID enteropathy (GI problems due to aspirin-like drugs)

- Chemotherapy-induced gut injury
- Pseudomembranous colitis

ENDOCRINE DISEASES

- Diabetes mellitus
- Autoimmune thyroiditis
- Obesity and metabolic syndrome

ALLERGIC DISORDERS

- Food allergies
- Skin eczema
- Asthma
- Nasal allergies

BACTERIAL INFECTIONS

- Cholera
- Helicobacter pylori in stomach
- Clostridium perfringens
- Clostridium difficile
- Certain forms of *E. coli*

VIRAL INFECTIONS

- Adenovirus
- Cox-Sackie virus
- Rotavirus
- HIV
- Hepatitis C

SKIN DISEASES

- Acne
- Psoriasis

- Rosacea
- Urticaria

LIVER DISEASES

- Alcoholic liver disease
- Intrahepatic cholestasis of pregnancy
- Nonalcoholic fatty liver disease
- Primary biliary cirrhosis
- Primary sclerosing cholangitis

RHEUMATOLOGICAL DISEASES

- Rheumatoid arthritis
- Lupus
- Ankylosing spondylitis

VASCULAR (BLOOD VESSELS) SYSTEM

- Edema or fluid swelling
- Endotoxemia
- Retinal complications of diabetes
- Hematogenous (blood-borne) spread of cancer

NEURO-PSYCHO-BEHAVIORAL DYSFUNCTION

- Emotional stress
- Autism
- Schizophrenia
- Depression
- Chronic pain syndromes
- Fibromyalgia
- Chronic fatigue syndrome

NEUROLOGICAL DISORDERS

- Multiple sclerosis
- Chronic inflammatory demyelinating polyneuropathy
- Parkinson's disease

MISCELLANEOUS

- Heart failure
- Parenteral or intravenous nutrition (Fasting patient obtaining nutrition via veins)
- Multi-organ failure
- Graft versus host disease
- Cancer and it's spread locally and metastasis to distant organs

Altered Genes or Phenotype May Lead to Gut Dysfunction Resulting in Different Syndromes

Based on expressed phenotype, different insults like inflammation and microbes can lead to *leaky gut* and variable disease manifestations.

Infections, drugs, toxins, inflammation damage tight junctions, activate mast cells and cytokines

Healthy gut

Leaky gut

Translocated bacteria, bacterial toxin along with cytokines increase stress hormones affecting central and peripheral nervous system.

REFERENCES

1. Zhang L, Cheng J, Fan XM. MicroRNAs: New therapeutic targets for intestinal barrier dysfunction. *World J Gastroenterol.* 2014 May 21;20(19):5818-5825.

2. de Punder K, Pruimboom L. The dietary intake of wheat and other cereal grains and their role in inflammation. *Nutrients.* 2013 Mar 12;5(3):771-87.

3. Lu Z, Ding L, Lu Q, Chen YH. Claudins in intestines: Distribution and functional significance in health and diseases. *Tissue Barriers.* 2013 Jul 1;1(3):e24978.

4. Ding L, Lu Z, Lu Q, Chen YH. The claudin family of proteins in human malignancy: a clinical perspective. *Cancer Manag Res.* 2013 Nov 8;5:367-75.

5. Fries W, Belvedere A, Vetrano S. Sealing the broken barrier in IBD: intestinal permeability, epithelial cells and junctions. *Curr Drug Targets.* 2013 Nov;14(12):1460-70.

6. Sawada N. Tight junction-related human diseases. *Pathol Int.* 2013 Jan;63(1):1-12.

7. Catalioto RM, Maggi CA, Giuliani S. Intestinal epithelial barrier dysfunction in disease and possible therapeutical interventions. *Curr Med Chem.* 2011;18(3):398-426.

8. Caricilli AM, Castoldi A, Câmara NO. Intestinal barrier: A gentlemen's agreement between microbiota and immunity. *World J Gastrointest Pathophysiol.* 2014 Feb 15;5(1):18-32.

9. Price DB, Ackland ML, Burks W et al. Peanut Allergens Alter Intestinal Barrier Permeability and Tight Junction Localisation in Caco-2 Cell Cultures. *Cell Physiol Biochem.* 2014 May 23;33(6):1758-1777.

CHAPTER 11

GI Diseases

KEY POINTS

- Diseases like irritable bowel syndrome, celiac sprue, and inflammatory bowel disease are associated with increased intestinal permeability.

- Exclusion diets tend to help in many of these diseases suggesting that some dietary component coming in contact with the body systems via leaky gut may be involved in causing or sustaining the disorders.

IRRITABLE BOWEL SYNDROME

FUNCTIONAL DISORDER

Irritable bowel syndrome, or IBS, is frequently labeled as a "functional disorder," and is being increasingly appreciated as an aberrant triggering of the immune system, causing low-grade inflammation in the gut.

EVIDENCE FOR LEAKY GUT

Dr. Park and colleagues from the Sungkyunkwan University School of Medicine in Seoul, South Korea studied a cohort of 38 patients with irritable bowel syndrome and 10 healthy controls. Subjects were administered polyethylene glycol (PEG) 3350 as the permeability probe. PEG 400 was given as a control. PEG 400 is a smaller molecule and normally absorbed by the gut and excreted in urine. PEGs 3350, on the other hand, is larger and poorly absorbed. The intestinal permeability or leakiness was found to be significantly increased in the patients with IBS compared to controls.

LEAKY GUT AND IMMUNE SYSTEM

Leaky gut facilitates an inappropriate activation of the intestinal immune system responses, resulting in IBS symptoms. The following facts support this hypothesis:

- There is increased intestinal permeability in patients with IBS.

- An increased number of immune-related cells are seen in the gut wall of IBS patients.

- Patients with self-reported food allergies have a higher prevalence of IBS and other allergic disorders. Allergies are associated with leaky gut. If IBS is associated with allergies, it would suggest that leaky gut is the common denominator.

- There is a subgroup of patients with IBS who have typical IBS symptoms in association with allergic symptoms; this may be called atopic IBS.

- IBS patients tend to have a high prevalence of chronic pain syndromes. In addition, they report multiple food allergies and intolerances. Exclusion of gluten as well as milk help symptoms in many cases.

CELIAC DISEASE

Celiac disease is an autoimmune disease caused by a toxic immune reaction to gluten contained in wheat, barley, and rye. Three factors involved in causing celiac disease are:

- Environmental spark (gluten from diet)
- Increased risk due to unhealthy genes
- Inordinate extent of gut leakiness

Celiac disease is a classic example where leaky gut is involved. There is an abnormal immune reaction, and a variety of organ systems of the human body are involved, causing variable clinical features in different persons.

The prevalence of celiac sprue appears to have sky-rocketed in recent decades. It tends to co-occur with many diverse autoimmune diseases suggesting a common underlying mechanism. Such diseases include:

- Microscopic and collagenous colitis

- Endocrine diseases like diabetes mellitus, thyroiditis, and Addison's disease

- Skin ailments like vitiligo, psoriasis, alopecia, and dermatitis herpetiformis

- Liver diseases like autoimmune hepatitis and primary biliary cirrhosis

- Rheumatological diseases like Sjogren's and lupus

How does it occur?

The gut barrier in celiac disease is leaky because of abnormal *tight junctions*, causing an increased absorption of unwanted material through the dysfunctional intestinal wall into the body. This permits gliadin contained in gluten to be absorbed, enter the body, and trigger an immune response.

- Alterations in functioning of some of the genes controlling *tight junctions* have been documented accounting for the abnormal structure of *tight junctions* in patients with celiac disease. The adjoining cells of the gut fall apart making it more porous.

- Intestinal permeability is increased in response to gluten in food.

- Abnormalities of the intestinal barrier are seen even in celiac disease patients without symptoms while on a gluten-free diet, suggesting that leaky gut is a cause and not an effect.

- Many healthy relatives of the celiac disease patients show evidence of leaky gut.

Celiac disease patients have varied symptoms beyond the gut, including liver disease. Such distant manifestations may be due to shared genes or the complex effects of abnormal intestinal leakiness, inflammation, and antibodies occurring due to the abnormal immune reaction.

Zonulin is a protein that is secreted by cells of the gut wall. This protein causes dismemberment of the tight junction. The more the zonulin in a person, the leakier the gut is likely to be. Gluten causes increased secretion of zonulin in patients with celiac disease making the gut leaky. This allows semi-digested gluten products to seep across the gut wall and interact with immune cells in the gut causing damage to the intestine.

Dr. Jauregi-Miguel and co-investigators from the University of the Basque Country in Spain have demonstrated that a gluten-free diet results in normalization of abnormal functioning of leakiness genes. Laboratory studies have shown that administration of probiotics reduces intestinal leakiness induced by gluten.

IMPROVED GUT LEAKINESS AS A MARKER OF RECOVERY ON A GLUTEN-FREE DIET

Exclusion of gluten from the diet forms the cornerstone of treatment. Drs. Ukabam and Cooper studied patients with celiac disease initially and then after several months on a gluten-free diet. 13 patients with celiac disease were studied as were 25 healthy controls. The Lactulose-mannitol test for intestinal permeability was done at baseline and then after 5-8 months of a gluten free diet.

The lactulose to mannitol ratio (L:M ratio) in celiac disease patients at baseline was significantly abnormal as compared to healthy controls. The L:M ratio or leakiness decreased in every patient after 5-8 months on a gluten-free diet. The L:M ratio normalized in 62% of the patients on a gluten-free diet.

INFLAMMATORY BOWEL DISEASE

Studies suggest that a leaky gut barrier is critical to the development of IBD (Crohn's disease and ulcerative colitis). The disrupted barrier results in an exaggerated immune reaction and inflammation. However, it by itself is not sufficient to cause IBD.

Dr. Dal Pont and colleagues from University of Padova in Italy suggest that testing for intestinal permeability should be used as a marker for disease activity in inflammatory bowel disease.

EVIDENCE FOR LEAKY GUT

Patients with IBD have abnormal *tight junctions*, making them discontinuous and leaky. In addition to an increase in inflammatory cells, there is an increased programmed cell death seen in the cells of the gut barrier.

- Experimental animal models of IBD first develop increased intestinal leakiness, which is then followed by the onset of colitis.

- Certain breeds of mice are prone to developing Crohn's disease. Increased gut leakiness in these animals can be documented before the development of Crohn's.

- Leaky gut can be seen in 35-70% of patients with Crohn's disease. 25% of first degree family members of patients with IBD have increased gut leakiness long before the onset of the disease.

Just a reminder that the available tests for gut leakiness are neither sensitive nor can test for all pathways or types of compounds that can pass through.

Dr. Katz and colleagues assessed the gut leakiness in 25 patients with Crohn's disease and compared it to controls. The Lactulose-rhamnose ratio in Crohn's disease patients' ratio was 70.5% as compared to 37.2% healthy relatives and 40.6% in unrelated controls.

PRESENCE OF LEAKY GUT MAY PREDICT RELAPSE

Dr. Wyatt and colleagues have shown that the presence of abnormal permeability test or leaky gut is 81% accurate in predicting the likelihood of relapse in patients with Crohn's disease. A case of a child with prior documented increased leakiness who developed Crohn's disease eight years later has been reported.

> IBD is associated with involvement of other organs like joints, liver, eyes, skin, etc. Mechanisms common to multiple organ involvement include an enhanced intestinal permeability. Drugs like Remicade that heal IBD not only suppress uncontrolled inflammation but also reduce the accompanying gut leakiness.

Studies indicate that patients with Crohn's disease benefit from limiting meat intake. Kids on a semi-vegetarian diet (80%-90% vegetarian) plus usual treatment tend to fare better as compared to a routine diet on similar therapy. This data indicates that some component of meat diet interacts with gut immune system via leaky gut thus sustaining the gut inflammation.

NSAID-INDUCED GUT DISEASE
(NSAID ENTEROPATHY)

Non-steroidal anti-inflammatory drugs (like aspirin and ibuprofen) cause damage to the gut. The damage can occur even if the drug is given by injection rather than as a pill. Increased gut leakiness is the central mechanism that converts the biochemical damage to tissue damage in the gut. Use of human lactoferrin (five grams per day for two days) by mouth diminishes the leakiness caused by the NSAID indomethacin.

REFERENCES

1. Piche T. Tight junctions and IBS--the link between epithelial permeability, low-grade inflammation, and symptom generation? *Neurogastroenterol Motil.* 2014 Mar;26(3):296-302.

2. Chang FY. Irritable bowel syndrome: the evolution of multi-dimensional looking and multidisciplinary treatments. *World J*

Gastroenterol. 2014 Mar14;20(10):2499-514.

3. Shulman RJ, Jarrett ME, Cain KC et al. Associations among gut permeability, inflammatory markers, and symptoms in patients with irritable bowel syndrome. *J Gastroenterol.* 2 2014 Nov;49(11):1467-76.

4. Jauregi-Miguel A, Fernandez-Jimenez N, Irastorza I et al. Alteration of Tight Junction Gene Expression in Celiac Disease. *J Pediatr Gastroenterol Nutr.* 2014 Feb 14.

5. Orlando A, Linsalata M, Notarnicola M et al. Lactobacillus GG restoration of the gliadin induced epithelial barrier disruption: the role of cellular polyamines. *BMC Microbiol.* 2014 Jan 31;14:19.

6. Mishra A, Makharia GK. Techniques of functional and motility test: how to perform and interpret intestinal permeability. *J Neurogastroenterol Motil.* 2012;18(4):443-7.

7. Juby LD, Rothwell J, Axon AT. Lactulose/mannitol test: an ideal screen for celiac disease. *Gastroenterology.* 1989 Jan;96(1):79-85.

8. Ivanov AI, Nusrat A, Parkos CA. The epithelium in inflammatory bowel disease: potential role of endocytosis of junctional proteins in barrier disruption. *Novartis Found Symp.* 2004;263:115-24; discussion 124-32, 211-8.

9. Dal Pont E, D'Incà R, Caruso A, Sturniolo GC. Non-invasive investigation in patients with inflammatory joint disease. *World J Gastroenterol.* 2009 May 28;15(20):2463-8.

10. Zeissig S, Bürgel N, Günzel D et al. Changes in expression and distribution of claudin 2, 5 and 8 lead to discontinuous tight junctions and barrier dysfunction in active Crohn's disease. *Gut.* 2007 Jan;56(1):61-72.

11. Lu Z, Ding L, Lu Q, Chen YH. Claudins in intestines: Distribution and functional significance in health and diseases. *Tissue Barriers.* 2013 Jul1;1(3):e24978.

12. Jenkins RT, Ramage JK, Jones DB et al. Small bowel and colonic permeability to 51Cr-EDTA in patients with active inflammatory bowel disease. *Clin Invest Med.* 1988 Apr;11(2):151-5.

13. Wyatt J, Vogelsang H, Hübl W et al. Intestinal permeability and the prediction of relapse in Crohn's disease. *Lancet.* 1993 Jun 5;341(8858):1437-9.

14. Katz KD, Hollander D, Vadheim CM et al. Intestinal permeability in patients with Crohn's disease and their healthy relatives. *Gastroenterology.* 1989 Oct;97(4):927-31.

CHAPTER 12

Liver Diseases

KEY POINTS

- Increased gut leakiness can be demonstrated in liver cirrhosis and many of its complications can be attributes to it.

- Chronic alcoholism may lead to alcoholic liver disease via its effects on intestinal permeability.

- Probiotics can ameliorate gut leakiness and decreases risk of liver disease in experimental models.

LIVER CIRRHOSIS

Liver cirrhosis is associated with increased intestinal leakiness as well as leakiness of the blood vessels. This leakiness can be documented prior to the appearance of DNA of intestinal bacteria in the patient's blood and body fluids. The increasing intestinal leakiness correlates with increasing severity of the liver disease.

Spontaneous infections of abdominal fluid (ascites) occur in such patients, likely due to the passage of gut bacteria across the leaky gut wall into the body. Antibiotics acting exclusively in the gut are frequently used in cirrhotic patients on an ongoing basis to prevent such infections further substantiating the concept that it is the gut bacteria that are responsible for such infections after crossing the gut barrier.

HEPATIC ENCEPHALOPATHY
(BRAIN DYSFUNCTION OF LIVER DISEASE)

Hepatic encephalopathy (HE) is more likely in patients with liver cirrhosis if they have small intestinal bacterial overgrowth as well. Symptoms of HE may be mild, such as altered behavior, confusion, slurred speech, and sleep problems, to more severe, such as sleeping much of the time, all the way to coma and unresponsiveness to pain.

Antibiotics that are poorly absorbed and work only on the gut are effective for the treatment and prevention of hepatic encephalopathy highlighting the role of gut bacteria and leaky gut in causing brain dysfunction.

The effects of liver disease on the brain are believed to be mediated via absorption of toxic substances across the leaky gut. Some liver societies recommend probiotics to manage this disorder.

ALCOHOLIC LIVER DISEASE

Alcohol causes damage to the intestinal wall, rendering the gut leaky. This, in turn, is one of the mechanisms involved in causing alcoholic liver disease.

- The toxin of the gut bacteria passes through the leaky gut into the body and causes inflammation, including in the liver.

- The increased bacterial toxin in the body also causes changes in the hormonal balance in the body. This increases the pressure in the veins of the stomach and esophagus. These veins can then rupture and cause life-threatening bleeding.

- Preventative use of antibiotics in liver disease patients with GI bleeding reduces the risk of death. This suggests that antibiotics are acting on intestinal bacteria that may be passing across the leaky gut wall.

FATTY LIVER DISEASE

Intestinal leakiness is involved as a factor in causing fatty liver disease due to obesity, drugs, toxins, alcohol, and other elements. Probiotic treatment with the beneficial *Lactobacillus GG* bacteria diminishes oxidative stress, intestinal leakiness, and liver damage in animals with fatty liver disease caused by alcohol.

PRIMARY BILIARY CIRRHOSIS (PBC)

PBC tends to co-occur with celiac disease. There is heightened intestinal leakiness in both disorders. The disrupted gut barrier exposes immune cells of the gut to the gut bacteria, and there is a subsequent immune reaction including antibody formation. This is evident from the fact that the anti-mitochondrial antibodies commonly seen in patients with PBC also cross-react with proteins from intestinal bacteria.

INTRAHEPATIC CHOLESTASIS OF PREGNANCY

Intrahepatic cholestasis of pregnancy (ICP) is a liver condition that may occur during late pregnancy and resolve after the delivery. Complications of ICP include damage to the growing fetus, still birth, and premature deliveries.

Key clinical features include:

- Pruritus (itching)
- Mild cholestasis (abnormal liver tests)

Dr. Reyes and colleagues from Chile compared the severity of gut leakiness in 20 ICP subjects with 22 normal pregnant women and 29 non-pregnant women. Intestinal permeability was higher in women with ICP, and these abnormalities persisted long past pregnancy.

The investigators concluded that leaky gut may be a factor causing this disease by increasing the passage of bacterial toxin from the gut into the woman's body, causing liver damage.

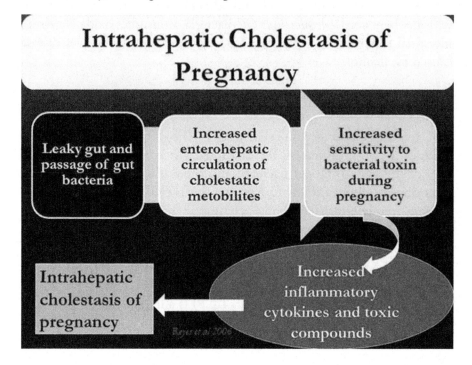

REFERENCES

1. Pijls KE, Koek GH, Elamin EE et al. Large intestine permeability is increased in patients with compensated liver cirrhosis. *Am J Physiol Gastrointest Liver Physiol.* 2014 Jan;306(2):G147-53.

2. Liboredo JC, Vilela EG, Ferrari MD et al. Nutrition Status and Intestinal Permeability in Patients Eligible for Liver Transplantation. *JPEN J Parenter Enteral Nutr.* 2013 Nov 19.

3. Zuckerman MJ, Menzies IS, Ho H et al. Assessment of intestinal permeability and absorption in cirrhotic patients with ascites

using combined sugar probes. *Dig Dis Sci.* 2004 Apr;49(4):621-6.

4. Dănulescu RM, Ciobică A, Stanciu C, Trifan A. The role of rifaximin in the prevention of the spontaneous bacterial peritonitis. *Rev Med Chir Soc Med Nat Iasi.* 2013 Apr-Jun;117(2):315-20.

5. Giorgio V, Miele L, Principessa L et al. Intestinal permeability is increased in children with non-alcoholic fatty liver disease, and correlates with liver disease severity. *Dig Liver Dis.* 2014 Jun;46(6):556-60.

6. Feld JJ, Meddings J, Heathcote EJ. Abnormal intestinal permeability in primary biliary cirrhosis. *Dig Dis Sci.* 2006 Sep;51(9):1607-13.

7. Di Leo V, Venturi C, Baragiotta A et al. Gastroduodenal and intestinal permeability in primary biliary cirrhosis. *Eur J Gastroenterol Hepatol.* 2003 Sep;15(9):967-73.

8. Reyes H, Zapata R, Hernández I et al. Is a leaky gut involved in the pathogenesis of intrahepatic cholestasis of pregnancy? *Hepatology.* 2006 Apr;43(4):715-22.

CHAPTER 13

Endocrine Diseases

KEY POINTS

- Mounting evidence points to the role of dysbiosis and leaky gut in diabetes and autoimmune thyroiditis.

- Use of probiotics has been shown to be helpful in diabetic animals.

DIABETES MELLITUS

FACTORS INVOLVED

The interaction of various discrete factors creates a "perfect storm" critical to the development of diabetes. Leaky gut, abnormal gut bacteria, an abnormal immune system, and abnormal genes appear to play a central role in causing diabetes.

A high fat diet induces increased passage of bacterial toxin across the gut into the body causing low grade inflammation.

ANIMAL STUDIES

Abnormal function of the gut barrier is seen in the *BioBreeding diabetes-prone rats*, which develop diabetes spontaneously on exposure to a normal diet. The altered intestinal barrier is seen in such animals prior to the onset of disease, suggesting that leaky gut is a cause and not an effect of the disease.

Administering probiotics to such animals reduces the amount of bacterial toxin as well as inflammation in the body and is associated with improvement of diabetes. These data suggest that gut bacteria can affect diabetes and the mechanism controlling the affects is leaky or strengthened gut barrier.

Tight junctions are abnormal with a widened space between the cells of the gut barrier in these rats. Levels of zonulin, the traffic conductor that regulates flow across *tight junctions* by opening up the passageways, are increased causing the barrier to be leaky. Zonulin blocking medications reduce diabetes in rats at high risk for diabetes.

Diabetics have decreased levels of proteins (occludin, claudin) interlocking the *tight junctions*. These proteins establish the *tight junction* seal between the cells lining the gut. Antibodies against pancreatic cells producing insulin may be present.

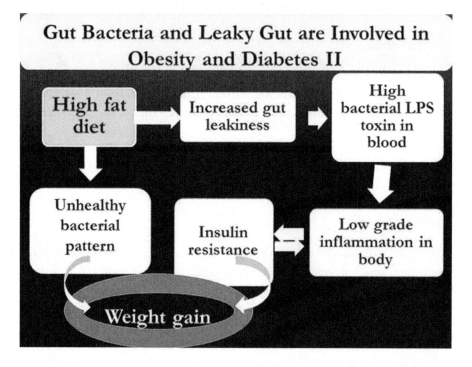

HUMAN DATA

Type-1 diabetes is common in patients with celiac disease and both disorders involve a leaky gut. Thus, leaky gut may be a common denominator in the cause of these two disorders.

- The gliadin component of gluten that is involved in celiac disease has also been implicated in type-1 diabetes.

- Prediabetic subjects with normal glucose levels show increased leakiness. The increase in leakiness is at the highest just prior to development of disease symptoms.

Many cases of type-1 diabetes are preceded by infection. Loss of intestinal barrier integrity by infection causes activation of the cells that cause diabetes. According to Dr. Skogg and colleagues of Uppsala University in Sweden, the rapid increase in diabetes argues against a critical role for genes. Rather, it suggests involvement of infectious agents or their breakdown products entering the pancreas, triggering the cascade to development of diabetes.

Breast feeding is known to strengthen the gut barrier and also protects against diabetes.

AUTOIMMUNE THYROIDITIS

GUT INFLAMMATION

There is the presence of low grade inflammation in the large intestine of patients with autoimmune thyroiditis. Inflammation in the gut causes it to be leaky. In addition, the disease tends to co-exist with other autoimmune disorders.

Studies by Dr. Bardella and colleagues indicate that autoimmune thyroiditis is the most co-existing disorder among ulcerative colitis, Crohn's disease, and celiac disease. They also stated that it may be related to these conditions having common causative mechanisms and altered intestinal permeability.

EVIDENCE FOR LEAKY GUT

Dr. Sasso and colleagues from the Second University of Naples in Italy performed the lactulose-mannitol test in thyroiditis patients and demonstrated that the gut is indeed leaky in these patients as compared to healthy controls.

REFERENCES

1. Campbell AW. Autoimmunity and the gut. *Autoimmune Dis* 2014;2014:152428.

2. Bosi E, Molteni L, Radaelli MG et al. Increased intestinal permeability precedes clinical onset of type 1 diabetes. *Diabetologia.* 2006 Dec;49(12):2824-7.

3. Neu J, Reverte CM, Mackey AD et al. Changes in intestinal morphology and permeability in the biobreeding rat before the onset of type 1 diabetes. *J Pediatr Gastroenterol Nutr.* 2005 May;40(5):589-95.

4. Cindoruk M, Tuncer C, Dursun A et al. Increased colonic intraepithelial lymphocytes in patients with Hashimoto's thyroiditis. *J Clin Gastroenterol.* 2002 Mar;34(3):237-9.

5. Sasso FC, Carbonara O, Torella R et al. Ultrastructural changes in enterocytes in subjects with Hashimoto's thyroiditis. *Gut.* 2004 Dec;53(12):1878-80.

6. Mori K, Nakagawa Y, Ozaki H. Does the gut microbiota trigger Hashimoto's thyroiditis? *Discov Med.* 2012 Nov;14(78):321-6.

7. Bardella MT, Elli L, De Matteis S et al. Autoimmune disorders in patients affected by celiac sprue and inflammatory bowel disease. *Ann Med.* 2009;41(2):139-43.

CHAPTER 14

Can't Lose Weight?
It's Not Just Wheat Belly!

KEY POINTS

- Dysbiosis, inflammation, and leaky gut barrier are involved in pathogenesis of obesity and metabolic syndrome.
- Probiotics in early life can help reduce the risk of obesity.

For the first time ever, overweight people outnumber average people in America. Doesn't that make overweight the average then? Last month you were fat, now you're average - hey, let's get a pizza!

—*Jay Leno*

ALTERED GUT BACTERIA

Intestinal bacteria stay in a balanced state through our lives despite instances of problems encountered intermittently. The evolving gut bacteria and intestinal barrier and its selective leakiness are inter-linked from early life. Such a bacterial resilience is lost in metabolic syndrome of obesity and diabetes.

INTESTINAL LEAKINESS

Intestinal bacterial and metabolic interactions play a critical role in increasing risk for obesity. A high fat diet creates abnormal bacterial balance in the gut that causes intestinal leakiness along with inflammation and insulin resistance. Increase in the passage of intestinal bacterial toxin through the leaky gut barrier in animals fed high fat diet triggers obesity, insulin resistance, and diabetes.

DIFFERENCES IN ENERGY HARVEST

There is also an increase in energy harvest from consumed food, causing low grade inflammation. Drs. Joyce and Gahan from the University College Cork in Ireland argue that gut bacteria, "impact upon the metabolic health of the host through pathways that influence satiety, gut permeability, and immune function."

ROLE OF EARLY LIFE EVENTS

According to Dr. Kerr and colleagues from Australia, "the effects of early life events on the gut microflora and permeability, whilst it is in a dynamic and vulnerable state, are fundamental in shaping the microbial consortia's resilience." Obesity itself also impairs intestinal barrier in a vicious cycle.

POTENTIAL INTERVENTIONS

Kerr and colleague also state that there are "potential interventions to recalibrate the 'at risk' infant gut microflora in the direction of enhanced metabolic health." An example is of *Flos Lonicera,* an herbal medicine used in Asia, which ameliorates obesity by controlling the distribution of intestinal bacteria and decreasing gut permeability.

REFERENCES

1. Kerr CA, Grice DM, Tran CD et al. Early life events influence whole-of-life metabolic health via gut microflora and gut permeability. *Crit Rev Microbiol.* 2014 Mar 19.

2. Teixeira TF, Collado MC, Ferreira CL et al. Potential mechanisms for the emerging link between obesity and increased intestinal permeability. *Nutr Res.* 2012 Sep;32(9):637-47.

3. Frazier TH, DiBaise JK, McClain CJ. Gut microbiota, intestinal permeability, obesity-induced inflammation, and liver injury. *JPEN J Parenter Enteral Nutr.* 2011 Sep;35(5 Suppl):14S-20S.

4. Wang JH, Bose S, Kim GC et al. Flos Lonicera ameliorates obesity and associated endotoxemia in rats through modulation of gut permeability and intestinal microbiota. *PLoS One.* 2014 Jan 24;9(1):e86117.

5. Horton F, Wright J, Smith L, Hinton PJ, Robertson MD. Increased intestinal permeability to oral chromium (51 Cr) -EDTA in human Type 2 diabetes. *Diabet Med.* 2014 May;31(5):559-63.

6. Joyce SA, Gahan CG. The gut microbiota and the metabolic health of the host. *Curr Opin Gastroenterol.* 2014 Mar;30(2):120-7.

CHAPTER 15

Joint Diseases

KEY POINTS

- Leaky gut is seen in many arthritic conditions including rheumatoid arthritis.

- Fasting improves symptoms of rheumatoid arthritis.

- Intestinal permeability is increased in ankylosing spondylitis.

- Antibodies against gliadin derived from gluten are increased.

ARTHRITIS

Joint diseases are linked to the gut in numerous instances. Arthritis is an extra-gastrointestinal manifestation of inflammatory bowel disease as well as certain types of infectious diarrhea.

Autoimmune antibodies against many joint diseases provoked by bacteria frequently arise from the gut. They attack joints recognizing them as foreign either because of cross-reactivity or mimicry supporting the concept that leaky gut is a key intermediate step in the causation.

Autoimmune disease producing pathways common to inflammatory bowel disease and various kinds of arthritis include not just autoantibodies against antigens seen in the colon as well as the outside gut, but also increased intestinal permeability.

EVIDENCE FOR LEAKY GUT

Studies performed by Dr. Smith and colleagues have demonstrated increased intestinal permeability or leaky gut in patients with rheumatoid arthritis. Studies from University of Alberta in Canada have corroborated these findings. Increased gut leakiness has also been documented to be increased in all types of juvenile arthritis.

Effect of fasting

Dr. Köldstam and Magnusson demonstrated that fasting for 7-10 days by well-nourished patients with rheumatoid arthritis results in relief of symptoms. Relapse occurs when eating is resumed suggesting that something in the food interacts with the leaky gut to enhance adverse immune-reaction.

Role of probiotics

Studies by Dr. Noto and co-investigators have demonstrated that the use of probiotic *Lactobacillus casei* fermented milk prevents reactive arthritis induced by *Salmonella* infection.

ANKYLOSING SPONDYLITIS

Evidence for leaky gut

- There is an increase in antibodies against gut bacteria seen in the blood of patients with rheumatoid arthritis as well as ankylosing spondylitis (AS) suggesting that these bacteria or their products enter the body to provoke an immune reaction.

- Other investigators like Dr. Fresko and colleagues have documented increased intestinal permeability in ankylosing spondylitis and lupus as compared to controls.

- Many patients with AS also show antibodies against gliadin derived from gluten.

- Studies from University of Edmonton, Canada have documented an increase in small bowel permeability or leaky gut in patients with ankylosing spondylitis.

- Dr. Martínez-González and colleagues from the University of Granada Hospital in Spain studied intestinal permeability in 20 patients with ankylosing spondylitis and compared it to healthy relatives as well as non-relative controls. The 51-Cr-EDTA resorption test was used. The intestinal permeability was increased in AS patients as well as their healthy relatives as compared to non-relative controls. The increase in leakiness bore no correlation with disease activity suggesting that the gut leakiness was pre-existing, and potentially a causative factor.

- Studies by Dr. Morris and colleagues using the 51Cr-ethylenediaminetetra acetate as a probe also documented similar increase in gut leakiness in AS.

WHY IS THERE DISCREPANCY IN TEST RESULTS SOMETIMES

Studies using the lactulose-mannitol test have not shown any link of AS with gut leakiness suggesting differences in sensitivity of the tests to detect leakiness.

REFERENCES

1. Yeoh N, Burton JP, Suppiah P et al. The role of the microbiome in rheumatic diseases. *Curr Rheumatol Rep.* 2013 Mar;15(3):314.

2. Rodríguez-Reyna TS, Martínez-Reyes C et al. Rheumatic manifestations of inflammatory bowel disease. *World J Gastroenterol.* 2009 Nov 28;15(44):5517-24.

3. Rashid T, Ebringer A. Autoimmunity in Rheumatic Diseases Is Induced by Microbial Infections via Crossreactivity or Molecular Mimicry. *Autoimmune Dis.* 2012;2012:539282.

4. Fresko I, Hamuryudan V, Demir M et al. Intestinal permeability in Behçet's syndrome. *Ann Rheum Dis.* 2001 Jan;60(1):65-6.

5. Picco P, Gattorno M, Marchese N et al. Increased gut permeability in juvenile chronic arthritides. A multivariate analysis of

the diagnostic parameters. *Clin Exp Rheumatol.* 2000 Nov-Dec;18(6):773-8.

6. Noto Llana M, Sarnacki SH, Aya Castañeda Mdel R et al. Consumption of Lactobacillus casei fermented milk prevents Salmonella reactive arthritis by modulating IL-23/IL-17 expression. *PLoS One.* 2013 Dec 10;8(12):e82588.

7. Holden W, Orchard T, Wordsworth P. Enteropathic arthritis. *Rheum Dis Clin North Am.* 2003 Aug;29(3):513-30.

8. köldstam L, Magnusson KE. Fasting, intestinal permeability, and rheumatoid Arthritis. *Rheum Dis Clin North Am.* 1991 May;17(2):363-71.

9. Toğrol RE, Nalbant S, Solmazgül E et al. The significance of coeliac disease antibodies in patients with ankylosing spondylitis: a case-controlled study. *J Int Med Res.* 2009 Jan-Feb;37(1):220-6.

10. Smith MD, Gibson RA, Brooks PM. Abnormal bowel permeability in ankylosing spondylitis and rheumatoid arthritis. *J Rheumatol.* 1985 Apr;12(2):299-305.

11. Vaile JH, Meddings JB, Yacyshyn BR et al. Bowel permeability and CD45RO expression on circulating CD20+ B cells in patients with ankylosing spondylitis and their relatives. *J Rheumatol.* 1999 Jan;26(1):128-35.

12. Morris AJ, Howden CW, Robertson C et al. Increased intestinal permeability in ankylosing spondylitis--primary lesion or drug effect? *Gut.* 1991 Dec;32(12):1470-2.

13. Martínez-González O, Cantero-Hinojosa J et al. Intestinal permeability in patients with ankylosing spondylitis and their healthy relatives. *Br J Rheumatol.* 1994 Jul;33(7):644-7.

SECTION III

Neuro-behavioral Dysfunction

CHAPTER 16

Autism

KEY POINTS

- Kids with autism display a greater immune reaction to food proteins.

- Absorption of biologically active partially-digested proteins across leaky gut can act on the brain and alter behavioral function.

- The *ScanBrit trial* has demonstrated that gluten-free, casein-free trial improves behavior function in autism.

I think that autistic brains tend to be specialized brains. Autistic people tend to be less social. It takes a ton of processor space in the brain to have all the social circuits.
—Temple Grandin

While many children with autism demonstrate increased gut leakiness, the involvement of gastrointestinal dysfunction in the pathogenesis of autism spectrum disorders (ASD) is mired in debate.

LEAKY GUT EXPLAINS BRAIN DYSFUNCTION

Leaky gut allows the bacteria, bacterial toxins, or large semi-digested food products in the gut to cross the gut wall and enter the blood circulation. These extrinsic compounds can then interact with the brain.

Dr. Theoharides and colleagues from the Tufts University School of Medicine in Boston suggest that non-allergic activation of intestinal and brain immune cells could provide unique targets for autism therapy.

DATA IMPLICATING LEAKY GUT IN AUTISM

Studies by Dr. Lau and colleagues from Columbia University have shown that children with autism have higher levels of antibodies against gliadin from gluten as compared to unrelated healthy controls. The underlying mechanism involves contact of normally unabsorbed gliadin with the body's immune system likely via a leaky gut.

Other lines of evidence include the following:

- One-third of patients with an ASD have a history of cow's milk and/or soy protein intolerance during infancy.

- Incomplete digestion of such dietary proteins results in absorption of semi-digested smaller protein components known as exorphins.

  o Exorphins are structurally similar to the body's own endorphins that are biochemically active in the brain.

- Both endogenous (endorphins) as well as exogenous compounds from food, etc., (exorphins) may act on the normally present opiate system in the body, especially the brain. Animal studies show that exorphins coming through the gut and into the body can reach the brain and can cause psychosis. Commonly identified exorphins include those related to gluten.

FURTHER EVIDENCE FOR LEAKY GUT IN AUTISM

- Increased reaction of immune system to food proteins.

- Greater degree of inflammation in the gut wall of autistic kids.

- Intestinal leakiness is seen in at least a subset of patients. Admittedly, the data is mixed. Again a reminder that the available tests for leaky gut are not sensitive and cannot assess integrity of all the possible passageways across the intestinal barrier. Gut permeability in ASD appears to be similar between ASD and special needs kids without ASD.

- GI symptoms are common.

SYSTEMS MODEL FOR REGRESSIVE AUTISM

Regressive autism occurs in apparently healthy kids at 15-30 months of age. Based on gut link to autism, Dr. Downs and colleagues from the University of Delaware have proposed a systems level model which indicates that altered gut bacteria along with inflammation increase intestinal permeability (leaky gut). This in turn precipitates the onset of autism.

This model highlights the importance of bacterial imbalance affecting distribution of bacterial neurotoxins in the body including different areas of brain.

EFFECT OF INCREASED PROPIONIC ACID

Their studies indicate that increased numbers of *Bacteroides vulgatus* bacteria in the gut cause a concentration of propionic acid. Injection of this neurotoxin has been shown to produce autism like behavior in rats. Enhanced immune activation provoked by intestinal bacterial imbalance produces inflammation and release of pro-inflammatory chemicals which make the gut barrier as well as the brain barrier leaky.

The leaky gut allows the proprionic acid to enter the body from the gut. The leaky brain barrier allows it to enter the brain and cause a neurotoxic damage.

THERAPEUTIC EVIDENCE

Studies including the *ScanBrit trial* have reported beneficial effects from dietary intervention with a gluten-free and casein-free diet. The autistic kids in the *ScanBrit trial* showed an improvement in communication, social interaction, inattention, and hyperactivity.

A *Cochrane database review* found that dietary intervention has significant positive effects on overall autistic traits, social remoteness, and overall ability to interconnect and interact.

Based on the aforementioned indirect circumstantial evidence cited, I believe that unhealthy gut and disordered digestion play a key role in initiating, exacerbating, and/or sustaining this disorder.

MULTI-DIMENSIONAL STRATEGY IS REQUIRED

Dr. Heberling and colleagues have proposed that a *"circular model"* is involved in causing autism. Multiple factors are involved. As such, treatments targeting one single factor may have limited utility. These authors proposed a multi-pronged treatment to target leaky gut, abnormal intestinal bacterial patterns, and metabolic defects as a treatment for autism.

REFERENCES

1. de Magistris L, Familiari V, Pascotto A et al. Alterations of the intestinal barrier in patients with autism spectrum disorders and in their first-degree relatives. *J Pediatr Gastroenterol Nutr.* 2010 Oct;51(4):418-24.

2. Souza NC, Mendonca JN, Portari GV et al. PG. Intestinal permeability and nutritional status in developmental disorders. *Altern Ther Health Med.* 2012 Mar-Apr;18(2):19-24.

3. Whiteley P, Shattock P, Knivsberg AM et al. Hooper M. Gluten- and casein-free dietary intervention for autism spectrum conditions. *Front Hum Neurosci.* 2013 Jan 4;6:344.

4. Galiatsatos P, Gologan A, Lamoureux E. Autistic enterocolitis: fact or fiction? *Can J Gastroenterol.* 2009 Feb;23(2):95-8.

5. D'Eufemia P, Celli M, Finocchiaro R et al. Abnormal intestinal permeability in children with autism. *Acta Paediatr.* 1996 Sep;85(9):1076-9.

6. Lau NM, Green PH, Taylor AK et al. Markers of Celiac Disease and Gluten Sensitivity in Children with Autism. *PLoS One.* 2013 Jun 18;8(6):e66155.

7. Catassi C, Bai JC, Bonaz B, Bouma G et al. Non-Celiac Gluten sensitivity: the new frontier of gluten related disorders. *Nutrients.* 2013 Sep26;5(10):3839-53.

8. Heberling CA, Dhurjati PS, Sasser M. Hypothesis for a systems connectivity model of Autism Spectrum Disorder pathogenesis: links to gut bacteria, oxidative stress, and intestinal permeability. *Med Hypotheses.* 2013 Mar;80(3):264-70.

9. Persico AM, Napolioni V. Urinary p-cresol in autism spectrum disorder. *Neurotoxicol Teratol.* 2013 Mar-Apr;36:82-90.

10. Kang V, Wagner GC, Ming X. Gastrointestinal Dysfunction in Children With Autism Spectrum Disorders. *Autism Res.* 2014 Aug;7(4):501-6.

11. McElhanon BO, McCracken C, Karpen S, Sharp WG. Gastrointestinal Symptoms in Autism Spectrum Disorder: A Meta-analysis. *Pediatrics.* 2014 May;133(5):872-883.014 Apr 28.

12. Goyal DK, Miyan JA. Neuro-Immune Abnormalities in Autism and Their Relationship with the Environment: A Variable Insult Model for Autism. *Front Endocrinol (Lausanne).* 2014 Mar 7;5:29.

13. Siniscalco D, Antonucci N. Involvement of dietary bioactive proteins and peptides in autism spectrum disorders. *Curr Protein Pept Sci.* 2013 Dec;14(8):674-9.

CHAPTER 17

Psychiatric Disorders

KEY POINTS

- Patients with depression have higher levels of antibodies against LPS toxin from gut bacteria.

- Injection of LPS toxin of gut bacteria can induce symptoms of depression.

- Probiotics have a beneficial effect in patients with depression and have been appropriately called psychobiotics.

DEPRESSION

Psychiatric factors may determine gastrointestinal health outcomes and vice versa. Intestinal bacteria and leaky gut play a role in depression. Evidence suggests that depression is associated with increased oxidative stress, inflammation, and an abnormally active immune system.

But where is this inflammation coming from?

Here is a clue. Injection of LPS toxin from gut bacteria into the human body can induce symptoms of depression!

A not well-appreciated fact is that intestinal bacteria also produce neurotransmitters in our guts. These include serotonin, melatonin, histamine, and acetylcholine. These neurotransmitters of bacterial origin communicate with nerve cells in the intestinal nervous system which then communicate with the brain and affects brain function.

Medications acting via serotonin are widely used as antidepressants. It should be noted that 95% of the body's serotonin is actually in the gut.

Intestinal bacteria ferment undigested food, producing several gases like carbon monoxide, hydrogen sulfide, and nitric oxide. These gases can also act as neurotransmitters.

For instance, when the brain is under stress, intestinal bacteria produce specific neuro-chemicals like putrescine, spermidine, spermine, and cadaverine.

An interplay of multiple discrete factors, like increased gut leakiness and increased inflammation with an abnormal immune system, compounded by stress can kick up a "perfect storm," leading to several symptoms of major depression involving multiple body systems.

Animal studies by Dr. Garate and colleagues have shown that chronic stress increases intestinal bacterial toxin in the blood presumably via passage across the leaky gut barrier. This activates Toll-like-receptors on white blood cells causing immune provocation which in turn results in behavioral depression. Use of antibiotics to kill intestinal bacteria blocks the stress induced increase in bacterial toxin in blood and inflammation in the brain.

Human data

Dr. Maes and colleagues examined whether an increase in the passage of toxins from intestinal bacteria across the gut and into the blood plays a role in causing major depression.

They found that the antibody levels to these bacterial toxins are much higher in depressed patients than those seen in healthy controls. The increase in antibody levels correlates with the severity of intestinal leakiness.

The above results suggest that disrupted intestinal wall function plays a role in causing inflammation and subsequent symptoms of depression (such as sadness, loss of energy, and changes in weight.) The authors suggested that such patients should be assessed for leaky gut by testing for an antibody panel and treated accordingly.

Studies conducted by Dr. O'Donovan and colleagues from the School of Medicine in Dublin, Ireland, have documented that suicidal thoughts in depressed patients are associated with increased levels of inflammation.

What is the source of this increased inflammation? Perhaps multifactorial but disordered gut, including dysbiosis and leaky gut, may be the key.

A fascinating human study

Dr. Keri and colleagues from the Budapest University of Technology and Economics, Budapest, Hungary took the animal studies by Dr. Garate a step further in an attempt to see if the same phenomenon of leaky gut and inflammation linked to depression occurs in humans. They also wished to see if there was a correlation with clinical symptoms.

These investigators studied newly diagnosed patients with major depression and compared them to controls before and after cognitive behavioral therapy (CBT) for treatment of depression. The investigators measured bacterial RNA as a measure of bacterial passage across the leaky gut barrier.

Toll-like-receptors (TLR) act as pattern identification sensors in cells including white blood cells. They play a critical role in detecting and recognizing bad bacteria or toxins and are the first to mount an immune reaction. The investigators also assessed the presence of inflammation occurring via TLR-4 pathway.

The results of the Keri study showed increased levels of intestinal bacterial RNA in the blood indicating passage of intestinal bacteria across the gut. There was concomitant increase in TLR-4 indicating activation of the immune system along with an increase in pro-inflammation markers like interleukin-6 (IL-6) and C-reactive protein (CRP). Most importantly, relief of clinical symptoms of depression as a result of CBT treatment was accompanied by reduction in TLR-4 levels.

MORE ON STRESS AND INTESTINAL BACTERIA

Intestinal bacteria not only affect the brain's response to stress but also the normal thinking function. The bacterial GABA neurotransmitter from the gut may impact the brain via the gut-brain axis. When harmful bacteria are introduced into an animal's gut, they activate the brain stem region, producing an anxiety-like feeling. Other bacteria, though, had the power to decrease anxiety in mice and enhance memory.

According to Dr. Berk and colleagues from IMPACT Strategic Research Centre, Deakin University in Geelong Australia, most of the factors involved in inflammation associated with depression are not carved in stone and are potentially modifiable. These include increased psychological stress, unhealthy diet, sedentary lifestyle, obesity, smoking, increased gut permeability, allergies, dental cavities, sleep, and vitamin deficiency, especially Vitamin D.

They argue that same factors may play a role in bipolar disorder, schizophrenia, autism, and post-traumatic stress disorder (PTSD).

MELANCHOLIC MICROBES VERSUS PROBIOTICS

The term "melancholic microbes" has been coined to describe the connection between unhealthy gut bacteria and depression.

Some data indicates that probiotics benefit psychological dysfunction. Dr. Dinan and colleagues from the University College Cork describe the term "psychobiotics" as the healthy bacteria of benefit in psychiatric illnesses.

Examples of psychobiotics include *B. infantis*. It produces gamma-aminobutyric acid (GABA), which is an important neurotransmitter involved in the regulation of anxiety and depression in the brain.

B. infantis administered to depressed animals normalizes their behavior. In humans, *B. infantis* is effective in treating irritable bowel syndrome by multiple mechanisms, including favorably modifying the ratio of pro-inflammation to anti-inflammation chemicals.

Reducing sugar in the diet improves behavior in some patients with depression. This probably happens through changes in gut bacteria resulting in altered fermentation patterns of sugars and production of different neuro-chemicals that can pass through the leaky gut.

GUT DISORDER MAY UNDERLIE CO-EXISTING DEPRESSION AND HEART DISEASE

Depression increases the risk for cardiovascular disease. Depression is 3 times more common in patients suffering a heart attack. Co-occurrence can be explained via a mechanism involving leaky gut.

UNHEALTHY GUT MAY UNDERLIE PTSD TOO!

Multiple studies have documented a higher level of pro-inflammation cytokines in patients with post-traumatic stress disorder. For example, Dr. Spivak and colleagues from the Ness Ziona Mental Health Center in Israel have demonstrated an increase in concentrations of interleukin-1 beta in persons with combat-related PTSD.

According to Dr. Gola and co-investigators from the University of Konstanz in Germany, PTSD is associated with increased spontaneous synthesis and release of pro-inflammation cytokines by white blood cells in the blood.

PTSD patients have a high frequency of GI disturbances including functional bowel disorders. It is therefore not beyond the realm of possibility that intestinal bacteria and leaky gut that are involved in other functional and inflammatory bowel disorders may play a key role in promoting a state of chronic inflammation in the PTSD body along with the resultant clinical manifestations in such patients.

SCHIZOPHRENIA

Autoimmune abnormalities and gut dysfunction have been linked to one another and to schizophrenia for a long time.

SCHIZOPHRENIA AND CELIAC DISEASE

Neuro-psychiatric dysfunction including schizophrenia is associated with celiac disease. Elimination of gluten from the diet can improve neurological symptoms in many cases.

EFFECT OF GLUTEN AND COW'S MILK

In addition to food allergies, many people are sensitive to wheat gluten and casein from the cow's milk. Casein also contributes to non-celiac food sensitivities in susceptible individuals. Concurrent gut inflammation, activation of immune system, and alteration in gut bacteria can be documented in many such cases.

Even immigrant status can be a risk factor. These comorbidities contribute to compromised gut barrier allowing the passage of otherwise non-absorbable semi-digested dietary proteins along with harmful bacterial components. The passage of such large molecules can produce conflicting and complex patterns of immune activation.

Drs. Genius and Lobo from the University of Alberta in Edmonton, Canada described a patient who achieved resolution of auditory and visual hallucinations upon elimination of gluten from the diet.

Dr. Severance and colleagues from the Johns Hopkins University School of Medicine, Baltimore, MD suggest that *"understanding of disrupted biological pathways outside of the brain can lend valuable information regarding pathogeneses of complex, polygenic brain disorders."*

REFERENCES

1. Raison CL, Lowry CA, Rook GA. Inflammation, sanitation, and consternation: loss of contact with coevolved, tolerogenic microorganisms and the pathophysiology and treatment of major depression. Arch Gen Psychiatry. 2010 Dec;67(12):1211-24.

2. Maes M, Kubera M, Leunis JC. The gut-brain barrier in major depression: intestinal mucosal dysfunction with an increased translocation of LPS from gram negative enterobacteria (leaky gut) plays a role in the inflammatory pathophysiology of depression. Neuro Endocrinol Lett. 2008 Feb;29(1):117-24.

3. Berk M, Williams LJ, Jacka FN et al. So depression is an inflammatory disease, but where does the inflammation come from? BMC Med. 2013 Sep 12;11:200.

4. Gárate I, Garcia-Bueno B, Madrigal JL et al. Stress-induced neuroinflammation: role of the Toll-like receptor-4 pathway. Biol Psychiatry. 2013 Jan 1;73(1):32-43.

5. Kéri S, Szabó C, Kelemen O. Expression of Toll-Like Receptors in peripheral blood mononuclear cells and response to cognitive-behavioral therapy in major depressive disorder. Brain Behav Immun. 2014 Aug;40:235-43.

6. Bested AC, Logan AC, Selhub EM. Intestinal microbiota, probiotics and mental health: from Metchnikoff to modern advances: Part II - contemporary contextual research. Gut Pathog. 2013 Mar 14;5(1):3.

7. Fetissov SO, Déchelotte P. The new link between gut-brain axis and neuropsychiatric disorders. Curr Opin Clin Nutr Metab Care. 2011Sep;14(5):477-82.

8. Severance EG, Yolken RH, Eaton WW. Autoimmune diseases, gastrointestinal disorders and the microbiome in schizophrenia: more than a gut feeling. Schizophr Res. 2014 Jul 14.

9. Genuis SJ, Lobo RA. Gluten sensitivity presenting as a neuropsychiatric disorder. Gastroenterol Res Pract. 2014;2014:293206.

10. Catassi C, Bai JC, Bonaz B et al. Non-Celiac Gluten sensitivity: the new frontier of gluten related disorders. Nutrients. 2013 Sep 26;5(10):3839-53.

11. Severance EG, Gressitt KL, Halling M et al. Complement C1q formation of immune complexes with milk caseins and wheat glutens in schizophrenia. Neurobiol Dis. 2012 Dec;48(3):447-53.

CHAPTER 18
Neuro-degenerative Diseases

KEY POINTS

- Leaky gut has been demonstrated in many patients. Low sensitivity of currently available testing techniques for intestinal permeability precludes accurate assessment of the prevalence of leaky gut.

- Levels of zonulin, a key traffic controller of gut barrier are abnormal in MS.

- Gluten-free diet may be warranted at least in those MS patients found to have gluten-sensitivity.

- Lewy bodies in brain are believed to be one of the first steps of the Parkinson's disease. The same Lewy bodies can also be demonstrated in the cells of the intestinal nervous system in these patients.

- Studies indicate increased gut permeability in Parkinson's disease.

Neurodegenerative diseases are widely believed to be precipitated by an environmental toxin that somehow enters the body and gains access to the brain. The type of illness depends on the type and severity of toxin/s and the vulnerable parts of the brain accessed depending on the genetic susceptibility.

MULTIPLE SCLEROSIS

Multiple sclerosis (MS) is an autoimmune disease affecting the central nervous system and is known to co-occur with other autoimmune diseases. GI symptoms are common in patients with MS.

MS AND GUT BACTERIA

The role of gut bacteria in pathogenesis of autoimmune diseases including MS has been gaining increasing attention in recent years.

Antibodies acting against intestinal bacterial antigens can be documented in many patients with MS, presumably a result of entry of these bacterial antigens through the gut barrier. Leaky gut can be demonstrated in at least a subset of patients.

TIGHT JUNCTIONS IN MS

According to Dr. Fasano from the University of Maryland School of Medicine, the levels of zonulin, a critical traffic regulator across tight junctions of the gut barrier, are increased in multiple sclerosis. This can explain the gut leakiness observed in MS and other autoimmune diseases. Passage of undesired bacterial, toxic, and semi-digested food products passing across the leaky barrier can then provoke unwanted reactions in different organs and cause disease.

GLUTEN SENSITIVITY

Data indicates that increased use of wheat and other gluten-related cereal grains could play a role in inducing chronic inflammation and autoimmune diseases. MS has been described as one of the extra-gastrointestinal manifestations of celiac disease. Gluten tends to increase intestinal permeability.

Induction of low grade chronic inflammation by gluten without a concomitant increase in intestinal permeability has been demonstrated in patients with irritable bowel syndrome. The latter suggests that our currently available techniques for testing intestinal permeability may not be sensitive enough.

There is a high prevalence of gluten sensitivity in MS patients. We need large, well-done clinical trials to examine the effects of a gluten-free diet on inflammation and gut leakiness in patients suffering from inflammation and autoimmune mediated diseases like MS.

According to Dr. Riccio from the University of Basilicata in Italy, "The control of gut dysbiosis and the combination of hypo-caloric, low-fat diets with specific vitamins, oligo-elements, and dietary integrators, including fish oil and polyphenols, may slow-down the progression of the disease and ameliorate the wellness of MS patients."

ROLE OF GLUTEN FREE DIET

Experts like Dr. Batur-Caglayan and colleagues from Turkey and Dr. Shor and co-investigators from Israel recommend that MS patients with GI symptoms should undergo investigations for gluten sensitivity, and those found to be gluten-sensitive should consider a gluten-free diet.

PARKINSON'S DISEASE

Parkinson's disease is widely prevalent and is the second most prevalent neurodegenerative disorder seen among elderly subjects. Gastrointestinal symptoms are common in Parkinson's. It was thought that such problems are a result of the disease. However, evidence from studies done in recent years suggests otherwise.

Complaints related to constipation and smelling dysfunction frequently predate the onset of disease by many years. Not surprisingly, the gut and the nose have been implicated as ports of entry into the body for the offending toxin/s.

LEWY BODIES OF PARKINSON'S ARE ALSO SEEN IN GUT

A key characteristic is the presence of an abnormal protein substance called Lewy bodies in the brain cells of these patients. Lewy bodies are believed to be one of the first steps of the disease that ultimately leads to the loss of brain cells.

Surprisingly, the same Lewy bodies as seen in brain can also be seen in the gut in such patients! In fact, these are seen in the cells of the enteric (intestinal) nervous system.

This finding has led to the tantalizing prospect that intestinal injury is the earliest problem wherein the gut is exposed to some toxin that may enter the body through a leaky gut. Once the body is exposed to such a toxin, it provokes oxidative stress and inflammation in cells of the nervous system and ultimately loss of neuronal cells.

LEAKY GUT IN PARKINSON'S DISEASE

Dr. Forsyth and colleagues from the Rush University Medical Center in Chicago, Illinois, studied a group of newly diagnosed subjects with Parkinson's and compared them to healthy controls. Multiple tests including urinary sugar tests to examine intestinal leakiness were done.

The investigators found that the urinary sucralose (marker of total intestinal permeability) excreted over the 24 period was almost twice the amount in patients as compared to age-matched controls.

LPS toxin is derived from gut bacteria. Low levels of LPS binding protein in blood are seen in subjects with leaky gut. In the *Forsyth study*, low levels of LPS binding protein were documented further confirming findings from the urinary sucralose test.

Colon biopsies showed the presence of an increased number of intestinal *E. coli* bacteria. These findings correlated with the severity of gut leakiness suggesting that passage of intestinal bacteria across a leaky guy may play a pathologic role in such patients.

REFERENCES

1. Shor DB, Barzilai O, Ram M, Izhaky D et al. Gluten sensitivity in multiple sclerosis: experimental myth or clinical truth? Ann N Y Acad Sci. 2009 Sep;1173:343-9.

2. Batur-Caglayan HZ, Irkec C, Yildirim-Capraz I et al. A case of multiple sclerosis and celiac disease. Case Rep Neurol Med. 2013;2013:576921.

3. Fasano A. Zonulin and its regulation of intestinal barrier function: the biological door to inflammation, autoimmunity, and cancer. Physiol Rev. 2011 Jan;91(1):151-75.

4. Fasano A. Leaky gut and autoimmune diseases. Clin Rev Allergy Immunol. 2012Feb;42(1):71-8.

5. Walker J, Dieleman L, Mah D et al. High prevalence of abnormal gastrointestinal permeability in moderate-severe asthma. Clin Invest Med. 2014 Apr 1;37(2):E53-7.

6. Vieira S, Pagovich O, Kriegel M. Diet, microbiota and autoimmune diseases. Lupus. 2014;23(6):518-26.

7. Yacyshyn B, Meddings J, Sadowski D et al. Multiple sclerosis patients have peripheral blood CD45RO+ B cells and increased intestinal permeability. Dig Dis Sci. 1996 Dec;41(12):2493-8.

8. Riccio P. The molecular basis of nutritional intervention in multiple sclerosis: a narrative review. Complement Ther Med. 2011 Aug;19(4):228-37.

9. Berer K, Mues M, Koutrolos M et al. Commensal microbiota and myelin autoantigen cooperate to trigger autoimmune demyelination. Nature. 2011 Oct 26;479(7374):538-41.

10. Berer K, Krishnamoorthy G. Microbial view of central nervous system autoimmunity. FEBS Lett. 2014 Apr 18. pii: S0014-5793(14)00293-2.

11. Berer K, Krishnamoorthy G. Commensal gut flora and brain autoimmunity: a love or hate affair? Acta Neuropathol. 2012 May;123(5):639-51.

12. Forsyth CB, Shannon KM, Kordower JH et al. Increased intestinal permeability correlates with sigmoid mucosa alpha-Synuclein staining and endotoxin exposure markers in early Parkinson's disease. PLoS One. 2011; 6(12): e28032.

13. Braak H, Del Tredici K. Nervous system pathology in sporadic Parkinson disease. Neurology.2008;70:1916–1925.

SECTION IV

Chronic Pain Disorders

CHAPTER 19

Distinct Pain Disorders or One Syndrome?

KEY POINTS

- Co-occurrence of poorly explained chronic pain disorders in the same individuals suggests that these are not primary disorders but part of an overall syndrome.

- Gut dysfunction appears to be a common denominator in many cases.

It is controversial whether the various chronic pain orders are distinct entities or represent varied manifestations of the same syndrome. Could it just be the bias of the specialty of the physician involved in the care?

Let's examine the issue of overlap since these chronic pain disorders tend to co-occur in the same individuals:

- Fibromyalgia occurs in 20-32 percent of patients with irritable bowel syndrome (IBS).

- 50-80 percent of fibromyalgia patients have IBS.

- A significant portion of charges for hospitalization for fibromyalgia patients are related to GI procedures!

- In one study, the overlap of IBS with other syndromes was 16 percent for TMJ disorder, 59 percent for fibromyalgia, and 36 percent for chronic fatigue syndrome.

- Multiple studies, including those by Dr. Chelimsky, indicate that interstitial cystitis is associated with other painful comorbid conditions like IBS, sleep problems, chronic fatigue, generalized pain, and migraine headaches. These co-occurrences mimic what we see in fibromyalgia and migraine.

The above data suggests these are not primary disorders but part of an overall syndrome with different names given based on the specialty of the physician seen.

ARE DIFFERENT DIAGNOSIS AN ARTIFICIAL SEPARATION?

DIAGNOSIS BASED ON SPECIALIST SEEN

Dr. Beard, a neurologist, wrote over 100 years ago about "neurasthenia," describing patients with fatigue, pain, and exhaustion. He suggested that these patients had GI symptoms, poor appetite, poor sex drive, and sleep disturbances. It sure sounds like he's talking about patients with fibromyalgia, chronic fatigue syndrome, and IBS.

Frequently, a patient is defined to have the disease based on the specialist he sees.

Dr. Wessley from the Guy's, King's and St Thomas' School of Medicine, London states that it is an artificial separation and that the diagnosis that represents the patient's view is the best diagnosis.

UNIFYING FACTORS FOR THE CHRONIC PAIN DISORDERS

- Pain-related disorders tend to occur in the same individual.
- Common mechanisms like functional brain changes and increased sensitivity to pain are seen.
- Therapeutic response to similar treatments is similar.
- All such pain disorders are deemed to be multifactorial, and the biopsychosocial model is invoked to explain diverse issues.

It appears that these pain disorders may just have different expressions of physical signs and symptoms to a varying degree, with some commonalities and similar mechanisms underlying pain disorder.

Altered brain activation patterns: A common theme is abnormal autonomic nervous system, which is connected to the brain at one end and other organs at the other end. This is likely related to abnormal incitement of the immune system.

An example is that of IBS wherein brain activity can be seen related to activated intestinal mast cells. Biochemical signaling molecules released by these cells sensitize the nerves and lower the pain threshold.

Immune activation may occur as a result of infection, abnormal intestinal bacteria, and food sensitivities in these disorders. Food triggers for worsening are seen in many patients. Elimination diets have been shown to be of benefit.

- Fibromyalgia is known to be preceded by infection, including various viruses and Lyme disease.

- There are similar reports of preceding infection in temporomandibular joint disorder (TMJD).

- An association with prior urinary tract infection is often reported in interstitial cystitis.

- Infections including viruses, bacteria, and mycoplasma have been associated with chronic fatigue syndrome. Post-infectious IBS is a well-described entity.

UNIFIED FRAMEWORK TO EXPLAIN THE UNDERLYING PROCESS

Different genes have been implicated in causation of various chronic pain disorders. However, these genes are likely multiple and contribute only a minor component to the overall disease process. Disease manifests when some other environmental factors come into play in the right setting of a "perfect storm."

The gut is the critical element for a unified framework. Inflammation, dysbiosis, and leaky gut can easily explain all the elements involved in chronic symptom-based pain syndromes and provide the basis for a unified framework.

- The process usually starts with an infectious GI problem, followed by post-infectious IBS. Added to that along the way are manifestations of chronic muscle pain, as in fibromyalgia and fatigue in chronic fatigue syndrome.

- The infectious agent disrupts the intestinal barrier, making the gut leaky. This exposes gut immune cells to the bacteria and their toxins. The result is inflammation.

- Bacterial toxins then migrate across the leaky gut into the body and gain access to the brain. Injection of bacterial toxin in animals produces flu-like sickness and fatigue.

REFERENCES

1. Martínez-Martínez LA, Mora T, Vargas A et al. Sympathetic nervous system dysfunction in fibromyalgia, chronic fatigue syndrome, irritable bowel syndrome, and interstitial cystitis: a review of case-control studies. *J Clin Rheumatol.* 2014 Apr;20(3):146-50.

2. Nickel JC, Tripp DA, Pontari M et al. Interstitial cystitis/painful bladder syndrome and associated medical conditions with an emphasis on irritable bowel syndrome, fibromyalgia and chronic fatigue syndrome. *J Urol.* 2010 Oct;184(4):1358-63.

3. Rodrigo L, Blanco I, Bobes J, de Serres FJ. Remarkable prevalence of coeliac disease in patients with irritable bowel syndrome plus fibromyalgia in comparison with those with isolated irritable bowel syndrome: a case-finding study. *Arthritis Res Ther.* 2013;15(6):R201.

4. Piche T. Tight junctions and IBS--the link between epithelial permeability, low-grade inflammation, and symptom generation? *Neurogastroenterol Motil.* 2014 Mar;26(3):296-302.

5. Friedlander JI, Shorter B, Moldwin RM. Diet and its role in interstitial cystitis/bladder pain syndrome (IC/BPS) and comorbid conditions. *BJU Int.* 2012 Jun;109(11):1584-91.

6. Othman M, Agüero R, Lin HC. Alterations in intestinal microbial flora and human disease. *Curr Opin Gastroenterol.* 2008 Jan;24(1):11-6.

7. Zhou Q, Verne GN. New insights into visceral hypersensitivity—clinical implications in IBS. *Nat Rev Gastroenterol Hepatol.* 2011 Jun;8(6):349-55.

CHAPTER 20
Chronic Fatigue Syndrome

KEY POINTS

- The levels of antibodies against the intestinal bacterial toxins are significantly increased in blood of patients with chronic fatigue syndrome (CFS). Levels of antibodies correlate with symptoms of CFS as measured on the *FibroFatigue* scale.

- Complexities associated with CFS suggest involvement of Gut-Immune-Hormonal-Brain axis.

MULTIPLE ASSOCIATIONS OF CFS

Evidence suggests that chronic fatigue syndrome (CFS) is associated with abnormalities of the immune system, along with increased oxidative stress and increased intestinal leakiness.

Besides fatigue, CFS is associated with multiple other problems like headaches, muscle and joint pains, difficulty sleeping, memory issues, difficulty concentrating, depression, and anxiety. Irritable bowel syndrome is more common.

MECHANISM OF DISEASE

Exact disease producing mechanisms have not clearly been established. High frequency of diverse problems suggests that the underlying defect cannot be in one organ i.e. brain.

More than likely, the underlying mechanisms involve a cohesive and integrated circuit of pathways inside the body such as Gut-Immune-

Hormonal-Brain axis or just simply brain-gut axis.

Disordered gut with underlying dysbiosis and leaky gut is being increasingly implicated in causation and/or persistence of CFS although conclusive evidence remains elusive.

According to Dr. Bested and colleagues from the Complex Chronic Diseases Program at BC Women's Hospital and Health Centre in Vancouver, Canada, "*It seems vital to underscore the fact that any discussion of microbiota and mental health, or probiotics as an intervention in behavioral medicine, is not akin to discussions*" of antidepressant drugs.

They argue that there are numerous ways in which the gut bacteria may interact with environmental factors, including the person's diet.

INCREASED ANTIBODIES AGAINST GUT BACTERIA

The prevalence and levels of antibodies against the intestinal bacterial toxins are significantly increased in patients with CFS as compared to normal volunteers. Levels of antibodies correlate with symptoms of CFS as measured on the *FibroFatigue* scale. This suggests that the gut bacteria and toxins enter the body through leaky gut and provoke immune reaction and inflammation. In fact, low grade inflammation plus increased pro-inflammation biochemicals have been documented in CFS patients.

ANTIBODIES AGAINST COW PROTEINS

The levels of antibodies against cow albumin in CFS patients also correlate with antibody levels against intestinal bacterial toxin suggesting that leaky gut allows the passage of cow's proteins as well as intestinal bacterial toxins into the body.

Leaky gut tends to increase the oxidative stress. Triggers of increased oxidative stress also provoke CFS exacerbation. These include psychological stress, sustained strenuous exercise, and viral as well as bacterial infections.

Normalization of leaky gut and levels of antibodies against the bacterial toxin in patients with CFS correlates with clinical improvement.

Drs. Ferraro and Kilman from the New York Psychiatric Institute said in 1933, "*We must not forget here the possibility that in the future more appropriate and more delicate biochemical methods may allow us to detect [circulating gut-derived toxins] in an easier and more accurate way than we are now able to do.*"

That has thus far remained a pipe dream!

Studies suggest that consuming beneficial bacteria (probiotics) reduces anxiety in patients with chronic fatigue syndrome.

Dr. Maes reported a case of a 13-year-old girl with CFS who showed very high levels of gut leakiness and inflammation. The patient was treated with antioxidants and put on a "leaky gut diet," resulting in normalization of the passage of bacterial toxin accompanied by a "complete remission" of the CFS symptoms.

REFERENCES

1. Groeger D, O'Mahony L, Murphy EF et al. Bifidobacterium infantis 35624 modulates host inflammatory processes beyond the gut. *Gut Microbes*. 2013 Jul-Aug;4(4):325-39.

2. Maes M, Kubera M, Leunis JC, Berk M. Increased IgA and IgM responses against gut commensals in chronic depression: further evidence for increased bacterial translocation or leaky gut. *J Affect Disord*. 2012 Dec 1;141(1):55-62.

3. Maes M, Leunis JC. Normalization of leaky gut in chronic fatigue syndrome (CFS) is accompanied by a clinical improvement: effects of age, duration of illness and the translocation of LPS from gram-negative bacteria. *Neuro Endocrinol Lett*. 2008 Dec;29(6):902-10.

4. Rao AV, Bested AC, Beaulne TM et al. A randomized, double-blind, placebo-controlled pilot study of a probiotic in emotional symptoms of chronic fatigue syndrome. *Gut Pathog.* 2009 Mar 19;1(1):6.

5. Lakhan SE, Kirchgessner A. Gut inflammation in chronic fatigue syndrome. *Nutr Metab (Lond).* 2010 Oct 12;7:79.

6. Maes M, Mihaylova I, Leunis JC. Increased serum IgA and IgM against LPS of enterobacteria in chronic fatigue syndrome (CFS): indication for the involvement of gram-negative enterobacteria in the etiology of CFS and for the presence of an increased gut-intestinal permeability. *J Affect Disord. 2007 Apr;99(1-3):237-40.*

7. Brenu EW, van Driel ML, Staines DR et al. Immunological abnormalities as potential biomarkers in Chronic Fatigue Syndrome/Myalgic Encephalomyelitis. *J Transl Med.* 2011 May 28;9:81.

CHAPTER 21

Fibromyalgia

KEY POINTS

- Intestinal leakiness is seen in patients with fibromyalgia.

- There is a high prevalence of small intestinal overgrowth which creates inflammation and increased intestinal permeability in fibromyalgia.

LEAKY GUT IN FIBROMYALGIA

Evidence supporting the concept of leaky gut in fibromyalgia comes from studies by Dr. Goebel and colleagues from the University Hospital in Wuerzburg, Germany. These investigators studied patients with fibromyalgia, patients with complex regional pain syndrome (See chapter 23), and healthy control subjects. Intestinal leakiness was examined using a standardized three-sugar test. The authors found that the intestinal permeability is increased both in patients with fibromyalgia and CRPS, compared to healthy controls.

CO-OCCURRENCE WITH SIBO

A high prevalence of small intestinal bacterial overgrowth (SIBO) which is known to cause inflammation has been documented in patients with fibromyalgia. The pain intensity of fibromyalgia correlates with the degree of small intestinal bacterial overgrowth, which in turn is associated with increased intestinal leakiness.

EFFECT OF GLUTEN FREE DIET

Many fibromyalgia patients experience improvement on a gluten-free diet suggesting that large semi-digested gluten breakdown biochemicals can pass through large pores in the gut and affect the body, further reinforcing the underlying concept of leaky gut in these patients.

REFERENCES

1. Goebel A, Buhner S, Schedel R et al. Altered intestinal permeability in patients with primary fibromyalgia and in patients with complex regional pain syndrome. *Rheumatology (Oxford)*. 2008 Aug;47(8):1223-7.

2. Isasi C, Colmenero I, Casco F et al. Fibromyalgia and non-celiac gluten sensitivity: a description with remission of fibromyalgia. *Rheumatol Int*. 2014Nov;34(11):1607-12.

3. Wallace DJ, Hallegua DS. Fibromyalgia: the gastrointestinal link. *Curr Pain Headache Rep*. 2004 Oct;8(5):364-8.

4. Zhou Q, Verne GN. New insights into visceral hypersensitivity— clinical implications in IBS. *Nat Rev Gastroenterol Hepatol*. 2011 Jun;8(6):349-55.

CHAPTER 22

Abdominal Migraine

KEY POINTS

- Triggers for pain include a variety of foods and fluids like fish and alcohol.

- It is believed to be a childhood presentation of those genes that later on in life may also be observed as precipitating migraine headache.

RECURRENT ABDOMINAL PAIN AND MIGRAINE

Patients with migraines are more likely to have chronic abdominal pain. Dr. Robbins from the Albert Einstein College of Medicine in Bronx, NY describes it as a "Cluster belly," a variant of irritable bowel syndrome. We have already discussed the role of gut bacteria and leaky gut in irritable bowel syndrome in previous chapters.

Frequent headaches occur in 50 percent of IBS patients as compared to 18 percent in the control population. Dr. Kurth and colleagues reported that 81 percent of migraine patients had GI symptoms as compared to 38 percent in the control population.

The concept of abdominal migraine is not unique. Similar to the pain of abdominal migraine, a syndrome of *abdominal epilepsy* is also well-described.

FEATURES OF ABDOMINAL MIGRAINE

- Diagnosed mostly in children but may be encountered in adults.

- Midline abdominal pain for one to 72 hours, usually without any headache, may occur in conjunction with reduced appetite, nausea, vomiting, and paleness. No other cause can be attributed to the symptoms, including no GI disorder.

- Pain triggers include foods like fish and alcohol.

- Strong family history of migraine headaches and motion sickness.

- Diagnosis is delayed by an average of six years.

- Refractory to usual medical treatments.

Childhood periodic syndromes are believed to be early life manifestations of those genes that later on exhibit migraine headache. Abdominal migraine needs to be considered in the differential diagnosis when recurrent abdominal pain associated with features of migraine is seen.

The prevalence of celiac disease in kids with abdominal migraine is high. While there are no direct studies examining the role of leaky gut in abdominal migraine, it remains plausible extension of the role of leaky gut in IBS and celiac disease.

REFERENCES

1. Teixeira KC, Montenegro MA, Guerreiro MM. Migraine Equivalents in Childhood. *J Child Neurol.* 2014 Oct;29(10):1366-9.

2. Dees B, Coleman-Jackson R, Hershey LA. Managing migraine and other headache syndromes in those over 50. *Maturitas.* 2013 Nov;76(3):243-6.

3. Evans RW, Whyte C. Cyclic vomiting syndrome and abdominal migraine in adults and children. *Headache.* 2013 Jun;53(6):984-93.

4. Carson L, Lewis D, Tsou M et al. Abdominal migraine: an under-diagnosed cause of recurrent abdominal pain in children. *Headache.* 2011 May;51(5):707-12.

5. Cristofori F, Fontana C, Magistà A et al. Increased prevalence of celiac disease among pediatric patients with irritable bowel syndrome: a 6-year prospective cohort study. *JAMA Pediatr.* 2014 Jun;168(6):555-60.

CHAPTER 23

Complex Regional Pain Syndrome or Reflex Sympathetic Dystrophy

KEY POINTS

- Precise cause of this painful disorder remains elusive.

- The bacterial pattern in the gut is abnormal showing reduced diversity.

- Increased intestinal permeability or leaky gut has been demonstrated.

CRPS/RSD IS KNOWN BY VARIOUS NAMES

Complex regional pain syndrome (CRPS) is known by a variety of different names like reflex sympathetic dystrophy (RSD), shoulder-hand syndrome, causalgia, reflex neurovascular dystrophy (RND), amplified musculoskeletal pain syndrome (AMPS), and Sudeck's atrophy.

The cause of the disorder is unknown and a variety of triggers have been identified. As of the writing of this book, RSD does not have any obvious nerve damage such as damage that can be seen in type II or causalgia.

Patients with CRPS/RSD have pain unrelated to issues involving chronic pain syndromes like fibromyalgia.

EVIDENCE FOR LEAK GUT

Dr. Goebel and colleagues examined intestinal permeability in patients with fibromyalgia using two sets of controls. They recruited not just healthy subjects but also patients with complex regional pain syndrome (CRPS) for comparison. The intestinal permeability or gut leakiness was increased in patients with fibromyalgia as they had hypothesized.

To their surprise, these investigators found that patients with unrelated pain disorder of CRPS also had increased gut leakiness as compared to healthy subjects and not different from patients with fibromyalgia.

ALTERED INTESTINAL BACTERIAL PATTERNS

Studies documenting alterations in intestinal bacterial patterns in CRPS (reduced diversity of bacteria) lend further credibility to the circumstantial evidence that gut is intimately involved in CRPS/RSD. Studies have suggested defective immune system involvement in causing and sustaining these diseases.

It is possible that the leaky gut allows for potentially toxic substances derived from diet or bacteria, etc. from the gut lumen to pass through the intestinal barrier. These toxins then interact with intestinal and extra-intestinal immune system as well as with nerve cells in the gut contributing to the disorder.

REFERENCES

1. Goebel A, Buhner S, Schedel R et al. Altered intestinal permeability in patients with primary fibromyalgia and in patients with complex regional pain syndrome. *Rheumatology* (Oxford). 2008 Aug;47(8):1223-7.

2. Reichenberger ER, Alexander GM, Perreault MJ eta al. Establishing a relationship between bacteria in the human gut and complex regional pain syndrome. *Brain Behav Im*mun. 2013 Mar;29:62-9.

SECTION V

Tentacles of Gut Dysfunction: A Potpourri

CHAPTER 24

Food Allergies and Asthma

KEY POINTS

- Healthy feeding practices during infancy can reduce the subsequent risk of allergies.

- There is increased intestinal leakiness in asthma.

FOOD ALLERGIES

Most cases of childhood food allergy do not persist into adulthood. In contrast, once a food allergy is established in an adult, it is rarely cured.

Leaky gut barrier allows abnormal/allergenic proteins from the food to cross the gut, inciting the immune cells in the gut wall to react and produce abnormal antibodies which start a war within the body.

Healthy feeding practices during early infancy promote the tolerance to different foods and reduce risk of allergies.

STEPS IN CAUSATION

- The initial critical step is interaction of the gut immune cells with the offending food protein through the disrupted or leaky gut barrier. The potentially harmful and/or poorly digested food protein passes between the cells of the leaky barrier into the gut wall and gains direct access to the gut's immune cells.

- The activation of the immune cells further disrupts tight junctions of the barrier, increasing leakiness in a vicious cycle.

- Once sensitized, increased leakiness persists, even if the offending food is excluded from the diet, suggesting that abnormal gut leakiness is a causative factor in food allergies.

FOOD ALLERGIES AND LEAKY GUT

Infants with a food allergy have increased intestinal leakiness as shown by the lactulose/mannitol ratio test for sugar absorption. The severity of symptoms is directly proportional to the severity of the disrupted gut barrier.

Food protein-induced enterocolitis syndrome occurs in kids up to age three. Usually, cow's milk and soy are the offending factors, although grains (rice, oat, and barley), vegetables, chicken, and fish may be involved.

Foods causing allergies can also trigger skin eczema. A defective skin barrier and defective intestinal barrier allow abnormal reactions to allergens to occur.

NEW ALLERGIES AFTER LIVER TRANSPLANTATION

Liver transplant patients have increased gut leakiness. The increased intestinal leakiness correlates with increased incidence of new food allergies starting in patients after the transplantation surgery. This occurs even if the donor of the transplant organ did not have a history of food allergies.

EOSINOPHILIC ESOPHAGITIS

Eosinophilic esophagitis (EE) is a disease of the esophagus involving some foreign antigen in the context immune dysfunction in persons with genetic predisposition.

Not unlike many other immune related disorders, the incidence of EE has been rising in recent years. EE is associated with celiac disease which is marked by increased gut leakiness.

The cause of EE has not been fully elucidated. There is an increase in eosinophil type of white blood cells in the esophagus suggesting an allergic reaction to a foreign allergen from the gut including possibly a dietary component.

Recent studies by Dr. Katzka and colleagues from the Mayo Clinic in Rochester, Minnesota, have documented an increased intestinal permeability or leakiness in patients with EE during active disease, and this leakiness is healed when the disease is in remission.

A *six-food elimination diet* helps many EE patients. Feeding kids an elemental diet with pre-digested food components also helps heal the disorder. Use of such elimination/exclusion diets suggest that the allergen coming in contact with the gut is derived from semi-digested food.

EE occurs less frequently in winter when there are fewer air-borne allergens suggesting that the offending antigen may also be derived from the environment.

According to recent data from Spain, most of the EE patients may need only a *four food group restriction* comprising of cow's milk, wheat, eggs, and legumes.

The above evidence suggests that the offending allergic substance, likely from the food, gains access to the body's immune system triggering an immune reaction causing the disease.

ASTHMA

INTERACTION OF GENE-ENVIRONMENT

Genes play only a minor part in causing asthma and an interaction of genes and environment is involved in causing and sustaining it. Allergies, pollutants, and toxins are involved.

While food and provocation by food additives and preservatives are key to only 6%-8% of patients with asthma, as many as 40% of patients with food allergies have respiratory problems.

ROLE OF GUT BACTERIA

Drs. Azad and Kozyrskyj point to the perinatal programming of asthma via the intestinal bacteria. Patients suffering from asthma have heightened intestinal leakiness as compared to patients with chronic obstructive pulmonary disease (COPD) and healthy controls.

Increasing data links obesity with asthma and the common underlying factor appears to be low grade inflammation, the source of which in many cases is through the leaky gut.

LEAKY GUT AND ASTHMA

A recent study by Walker and co-investigators reported in the journal *Clinical Investigative Medicine* (2014) found that as many as half of the patients with moderate-severe asthma have increased gastrointestinal permeability or leakiness.

The authors concluded that leaky gut may be separately or sequentially involved with the development and persistence of asthma over the long term.

The results of Walker study results are in line with a report from Drs. Dunlop and colleagues who showed that IBS patients with eczema or asthma have increases in intestinal leakiness as compared to IBS subjects without atopy.

ASTHMA AND GUT IMMUNE SYSTEM

Boosting airway immune cells by stimulation of intestinal immune cells has been advocated as a strategy for better control of asthma.

Dr. Nekam from the National Institute of Rheumatology in Budapest, Hungary, argues for the avoidance of food triggers in conjunction with measures to reduce intestinal permeability.

REFERENCES

1. Järvinen KM, Konstantinou GN, Pilapil M et al. Intestinal permeability in children with food allergy on specific elimination diets. *Pediatr Allergy Immunol.* 2013 Sep;24(6):589-95.

2. Perrier C, Corthésy B. Gut permeability and food allergies. *Clin Exp Allergy.* 2011 Jan;41(1):20-8.

3. Yu LC. The epithelial gatekeeper against food allergy. *Pediatr Neonatol.* 2009 Dec;50(6):247-54.

4. Katzka DA, Geno DM, Blair HE et al. Small intestinal permeability in patients with eosinophilic oesophagitis during active phase and remission. *Gut.* 2014 Jun 23.

5. WalkermJ, Dieleman L, Mah D et al. High prevalence of abnormal gastrointestinal permeability in moderate-severe asthma. *Clin Invest Med.* 2014 Apr 1;37(2):E53-7.

6. Benard A, Desreumeaux P, Huglo D et al. Increased intestinal permeability in bronchial asthma. *J Allergy Clin Immunol.* 1996 Jun;97(6):1173-8.

7. Azad MB, Kozyrskyj AL. Perinatal programming of asthma: the role of gut microbiota. *Clin Dev Immunol.* 2012;2012:932072.

8. Nékám KL. Nutritional triggers in asthma. *Acta Microbiol Immunol Hung.*1998;45(1):113-7.

9. Gillman A, Douglass JA. What do asthmatics have to fear from food and additive allergy? *Clin Exp Allergy.* 2010 Sep;40(9):1295-302.

10. Dunlop SP, Hebden J, Campbell E et al. Abnormal intestinal permeability in subgroups of diarrhea-predominant irritable bowel syndromes. *Am J Gastroenterol.* 2006 Jun;101(6):1288-94.

11. Price DB, Ackland ML, Burks W, Knight MI, Suphioglu C. Peanut Allergens Alter Intestinal Barrier Permeability and Tight Junction Localisation in Caco-2 Cell Cultures. *Cell Physiol Biochem.* 2014 May 23;33(6):1758-1777.

CHAPTER 25

Skin Diseases

KEY POINTS

- Many skin diseases tend to co-occur with some GI diseases.
- Gut-skin-immune-brain axis has been implicated in causation of many poorly explained skin diseases via leaky gut mechanisms.

Glamour is about feeling good in your own skin.
—Zoe Saldana

The co-occurrence of skin diseases like eczema and psoriasis, etc., as well as joint diseases with small intestinal abnormalities has been reported for a long time.

For example, Dr. Paganelli and colleagues reported decades ago that intestinal permeability is increased in patients with chronic urticaria (hives) as well as joint problems.

In fact, they recommended screening certain subtypes of subjects for the leaky gut in order to identify patients who might benefit from elimination diets.

GUT-SKIN-IMMUNE-BRAIN AXIS

A gut-skin-immune-brain axis is believed to be part of this inter-organ communication system, as both the gut and the skin demonstrate comparable nerve messaging and inflammation related activities.

The existence of such communication axis has been proven in animals. Use of probiotics by mouth has been shown to improve stress-induced neurogenic inflammation of the skin. Based on these animal experiments, it is reasonable to assume that a similar inter-connected network exists in humans.

SKIN ECZEMA OR ATOPIC DERMATITIS

An intestinal barrier dysfunction appears to play a key role by allowing migration of harmful antigen through the broken gut barrier. Allergic sensitization appears to be preceded by changes in the person's unique fingerprint of his/her distinctive gut bacterial pattern.

Disruption of both the skin and intestinal barrier are involved. There is the potential for passage of unhealthy food antigens in persons with unhealthy genes during periods of increased permeability like acute sickness.

Increased immune complexes containing food proteins as foreign substances are seen in atopic subjects. This can lead to skin diseases, including skin allergies.

Symptoms may sometimes occur within minutes of consuming food, without any skin eczema itself. Some patients suffer from worsening of skin eczema with certain food triggers.

There is variability of skin eczema based on immune reactions to respiratory and food borne allergenic triggers further endorsing the key role of the gut.

Probiotics can help treat skin eczema. Multiple studies have documented the beneficial effect of probiotics in reversing the increased intestinal leakiness and reducing the risk of skin eczema in high-risk infants whose parents have history of allergies.

ACNE

Increasing evidence suggests that abnormal intestinal bacteria and leaky gut are involved in causing and/or perpetuating or exacerbating acne.

According to the gut-brain-skin axis theory, the use of probiotics for healing is based on their effect on mental depression, anxiety, inflammation, oxidative stress, body fat and even mood and temperament.

According to Dr. Bowe and colleagues from the State University of New York Downstate Medical Center in Brooklyn, NY, "*This intricate relationship between gut microbiota and the skin may also be influenced by diet.*"

Drs. Tremellen and Pearce from Australia argue that leaky gut is the underlying mechanism responsible for polycystic syndrome and its associated acne.

PSORIASIS

Abnormalities of intestinal structure and function have been implicated in causing psoriasis. Genetic abnormalities known to be risk factors for gastrointestinal diseases (inflammatory bowel disease, celiac disease) are also related to psoriasis.

Likewise, abnormalities of *tight junctions* of the intestinal wall are seen not only in inflammatory bowel disease but also in some types of psoriasis.

- Microscopic abnormalities of the colon are seen in patients with psoriasis, even when the intestinal wall appears normal to the naked eye.

- Psoriasis is common in patients with celiac disease which is known to have leaky gut.

Dr. Humbert and colleagues studied intestinal permeability in psoriatic patients and healthy controls using the EDTA absorption test. The 24-

hour urine excretion of EDTA from psoriatic patients was significantly higher than in controls, suggesting that leaky gut is present.

ROSACEA

The cause of rosacea continues to defy science. Patients tend to have a higher prevalence of GI problems. In addition, rosacea is associated with GI diseases known to have manifestations beyond the gut, e.g. inflammatory bowel disease and celiac disease. Stomach infection with *Helicobacter pylori* bacteria has also been observed.

Disordered gut including altered intestinal bacterial pattern has been implicated in the causation of rosacea via the gut-immune-skin-brain axis. Abnormal stimulation of the immune system appears to be involved in rosacea.

Such a stimulation may be due to a bacteria whether in the gut or on the skin. The dysbiosis may affect rosacea via multiple mechanisms including, but not limited to, leaky gut that can be caused and perpetuated by unhealthy bacteria.

Small intestinal bacterial overgrowth (SIBO) is associated with gut inflammation and leakiness. Dr. Parody and colleagues from the University of Genoa, Italy wanted to examine the role of SIBO in the causation of rosacea. They studied 113 rosacea patients and 60 healthy age-sex matched controls. 46 percent of rosacea patients had SIBO as compared to only 5% among healthy controls. Of the patients in whom SIBO was effectively eradicated, 71% of the patients totally cleared the rosacea lesions whereas 21% were greatly improved. Another recent study from the Washington University School of Medicine, found the prevalence of SIBO to be 51% as compared to 10% in completely healthy subjects.

Relief of rosacea using the antibiotics working solely in the gut strongly link the gut and skin together in causation. Probiotics have been used to effectively treat SIBO.

Perhaps, we should use probiotics to treat rosacea. Limited data suggest that *Lactobacillus casei Shirota* as well as a blend of *Lactobacillus casei, Lactobacillus plantarum, Streptococcus faecalis,* and *Bifidobacterium brevis* are effective in eradicating SIBO.

Some dermatologists are already prescribing probiotics as an adjunct treatment of skin disorders like acne and rosacea.

Dr. Kendall from the University of Warwick in the UK reported a case of a rosacea patient with constipation and increased gut leakiness who was given wheat bran agents to "flush" the gut. The wheat bran produced significant increase in frequency of bowel movements along with beneficial effect on rosacea. The relief was associated with concurrent relief of the patient's migraine headaches. The author speculated that such a treatment may also be of benefit in fibromyalgia and some psychiatric disorders.

URTICARIA

Urticaria, or hives, is a complex syndrome that affects as many as 20% of the people at some time during their lives. Both immune and non-immune pathways may be involved. Leaky gut has been implicated. Food allergens are involved in many cases which supports the leaky gut as an underlying factor.

A broken gut barrier allows undesirable antigens to pass through the gut creating antibody formation that cause degranulation of mast cells and symptoms. Urticaria tends to co-occur in patients with other autoimmune diseases like thyroiditis. Cow's milk allergy can induce urticaria.

REFERENCES

1. Drago L, Toscano M, Pigatto PD. Probiotics: immunomodulatory properties in allergy and eczema. *G Ital Dermatol Venereol.* 2013 Oct;148(5):505-14.

2. Kalliomäki M, Isolauri E. Pandemic of atopic diseases--a lack of microbial exposure in early infancy? *Curr Drug Targets Infect Disord.* 2002 Sep;2(3):193-9.

3. Pike MG, Heddle RJ, Boulton P et al. Increased intestinal permeability in atopic eczema. *J Invest Dermatol.* 1986 Feb;86(2):101-4.

4. Rosenfeldt V, Benfeldt E, Valerius NH et al. Effect of probiotics on gastrointestinal symptoms and small intestinal permeability in children with atopic dermatitis. *J Pediatr.* 2004 Nov;145(5):612-6.

5. Fabrizi G, Romano A, Vultaggio P et al. Heterogeneity of atopic dermatitis defined by the immune response to inhalant and food allergens. *Eur J Dermatol.* 1999 Jul-Aug;9(5):380-4.

6. Paganelli R, Fagiolo U, Cancian M, Scala E. Intestinal permeability in patients with chronic urticaria-angioedema with and without arthralgia. *Ann Allergy.* 1991 Feb;66(2):181-4.

7. Tremellen K, Pearce K. Dysbiosis of Gut Microbiota (DOGMA)--a novel theory for the development of Polycystic Ovarian Syndrome. *Med Hypotheses.* 2012 Jul;79(1):104-12.

8. Asero R. Hypersensitivity to lipid transfer protein is frequently associated with chronic urticaria. *Eur Ann Allergy Clin Immunol.* 2011 Feb;43(1):19-21

9. Sicherer SH. Determinants of systemic manifestations of food allergy. *J Allergy Clin Immunol.* 2000 Nov;106(5 Suppl):S251-7.

CHAPTER 26

Miscellaneous

KEY POINTS

- Leaky gut has been implicated as a causative or worsening factor in a variety of other diseases including severe pancreatitis, cancer spread, AIDS, aging-associated dementia, heart failure, sepsis syndrome, and multi-organ failure.

- Abnormal structure and reduced number of *tight junctions* are involved in cancer.

CANCER

Leaky gut increases the risk for cancer including its spread via multiple mechanisms including:

- Decrease in or loss of *tight junctions* causing loosened linkages in barrier.

- Altered components of *tight junctions* like claudin proteins creating a loosened dysfunctional barrier.

Chronic constipation patients demonstrate different gut bacteria than controls. The stool stasis can allow for build-up of potentially toxic compounds that in turn can create low grade inflammation and cause the gut to be leaky. For example, a study of over 115,000 patients demonstrated that subjects suffering from chronic constipation are more likely to develop colon polyps and cancer. The increased risk correlates with the severity of constipation.

Leaky gut has also been implicated in causing the complications of treatment of cancer including surgery and chemotherapy.

Multiple studies have documented the benefit of probiotics in reducing the risk of cancer recurrence in patients with transitional cell type of cancer of the bladder following resection. One of the mechanisms of actions of probiotics is strengthening the leaky gut barrier.

HIV INFECTION AND AIDS

Increased gut permeability is seen in HIV infection. Passage of intestinal bacteria or their products across the gut wall occurs, as demonstrated by increased levels of intestinal bacterial toxin in the blood. The levels decline in patients on anti-HIV treatment.

Dr. Leite and colleagues conducted a randomized, controlled trial and found that glutamine administration helps improve intestinal permeability problems in HIV patients.

AGING-ASSOCIATED DEMENTIA

Elderly patients may suffer increased leakiness due to impaired blood flow and the increased use of gut-toxic medications, especially aspirin, ibuprofen-like drugs known as NSAIDs. Some experts have speculated that this may contribute to cognitive decline.

While controlled data of aging in humans shows no differences in usual intestinal parameters, data from animals suggests otherwise. Puppies and large dogs have higher intestinal permeability than adult and small dogs.

According to Dr. Brenner at the St. Louis Veterans Affairs Medical Center, a leaky gut would allow intestinal contents to go across the gut wall into the body. They may then reach the brain via the blood and create abnormalities of brain cells and cognitive decline.

CONGESTIVE HEART FAILURE (CHF)

CHF is being increasingly recognized as a disease involving multiple organ systems in the body. Mechanisms include hormonal imbalance and increased gut leakiness.

Dr. Sandek and colleagues studied 22 patients with CHF and compared them to healthy controls. They found a 35 percent increase in gut leakiness in CHF patients.

The disruption of the intestinal barrier results in increased passage of intestinal bacterial toxins into the body. This, in turn, causes inflammation, which further worsens heart dysfunction.

As noted previously, inflammatory bowel disease (IBD) is a classic example of leaky gut. A study presented at the Heart Failure Congress 2014 demonstrated that patients with IBD have two and half times the increased risk of being hospitalized due to flare ups of their heart failure.

The above evidence suggests that intestinal dysfunction and leaky intestinal barrier may underlie the chronic low-grade inflammation and the resulting malnutrition in CHF patients. The gut offers an attractive target for therapeutic interventions in congestive heart failure.

References

1. Rera M, Clark RI, Walker DW. Intestinal barrier dysfunction links metabolic and inflammatory markers of aging to death in Drosophila. *Proc Natl Acad Sci U SA*. 2012 Dec 26;109(52):21528-33.

2. Catalioto RM, Maggi CA, Giuliani S. Intestinal epithelial barrier dysfunction in disease and possible therapeutical interventions. *Curr Med Chem*. 2011;18(3):398-426.

3. Mishra A, Makharia GK. Techniques of functional and motility test: how to perform and interpret intestinal permeability. *J Neurogastroenterol Motil.* 2012 Oct;18(4):443-7.

4. Klein GL, Petschow BW, Shaw AL et al. Gut barrier dysfunction and microbial translocation in cancer cachexia: a new therapeutic target. *Curr Opin Support Palliat Care.* 2013 Dec;7(4):361-7.

5. Carvalho BM, Saad MJ. Influence of gut microbiota on subclinical inflammation and insulin resistance. *Mediators Inflamm.* 2013;2013:986734.

6. Wardill HR, Bowen JM, Gibson RJ. Chemotherapy-induced gut toxicity: are alterations to intestinal tight junctions pivotal? *Cancer Chemother Pharmacol.* 2012 Nov;70(5):627-35.

SECTION VI

What if You Suspect Leaky Gut

CHAPTER 27

Testing for Leaky Gut

KEY POINTS

- There are limitations to current laboratory techniques available for testing for leaky gut.

- Testing for leaky gut is not widely available.

- Screening for leaky gut has been recommended by a few experts for patients at high risk of autoimmune diseases.

The trouble with the world is that the stupid are cocksure
and the intelligent full of doubt.
—*Bertrand Russell*

Testing for gut permeability is not a recent discovery. The first report of such testing from Dr. Fordtran and colleagues was published in the *Journal of Clinical Investigation* in 1965. Dr. Menzies was the first to use the sugar molecules for testing intestinal permeability.

The gut has pores of various sizes. While smaller compounds can be absorbed through smaller pores, larger ones are limited by having to use larger pores that are less accessible and also fewer in number. Leaky gut primarily implies passage across the gut of substances larger than molecular weight of 150 Da.

Current testing techniques depend on many factors and as such have pitfalls. They are also limited by the fact that we are only able to assess passage of water soluble compounds but not the fat soluble substances! In addition, the widely used sugar tests cannot account for passage of semi-digested proteins, bacteria, and its toxins.

155

SUGAR-BASED TESTS

The sugar combinations of lactulose with mannitol and lactulose/ rhamnose measure small intestinal permeability, while 51Cr-EDTA/ mannitol, sucralose with mannitol, and sucralose with rhamnose are useful to measure the overall permeability of entire gut.

Lactulose-mannitol test

While the smaller mannitol sugar utilizes the numerous small pores or *tight junctions* in the gut for its passage with impunity, lactulose, because of its larger size, requires the larger pores and as such is not well absorbed.

If the gut permeability is increased, i.e., leaky gut, more of the large and otherwise non-absorbable substance like lactulose is absorbed into the body and appears in the urine.

INDIRECT TESTS

Leaky gut allows for passage of bacteria and/or its component toxins which then come into contact with the body's immune system. Such a contact provokes formation of antibodies which can then be measured in blood. An example is testing for antibodies directed against LPS toxin of intestinal bacteria.

SCREENING FOR LEAKY GUT

Should we test and screen?

The testing and screening is not routinely recommended.

- Tests are not widely available.
- Tests are not sensitive enough.
- Effect of testing on outcomes remains unclear.

POTENTIAL CANDIDATES FOR SCREENING

Drs. Mishra and Makharia from the AIIMS in New Delhi, India have suggested the use of permeability testing to check for increase in risk for certain autoimmune diseases. A similar recommendation for testing has been made by Dr. Maes arguing for testing for antibody against intestinal bacterial toxin and if positive, to be treated accordingly.

A SUCCESSFUL STORY

Success of the screening strategy bearing fruit was reported by Drs. Irvine and Marshall from the McMaster University, Hamilton, Ontario, Canada. A child found to have leaky gut during screening of family members of patients with Crohn's disease demonstrated the onset of Crohn's disease 8 years later.

REFERENCES

1. Mishra A, Makharia GK. Techniques of functional and motility test: how to perform and interpret intestinal permeability. *J Neurogastroenterol Motil.* 2012 Oct;18(4):443-7.

2. Salles Teixeira TF, Boroni Moreira AP, Silva Souza NC et al. Intestinal permeability measurements: general aspects and possible pitfalls. *Nutr Hosp.* 2014 Feb 1;29(2):269-81.

3. Vojdani A. For the assessment of intestinal permeability, size matters. *Altern Ther Health Med.* 2013 Jan-Feb;19(1):12-24.

4. Fordtran JS, Rector FC, Ewton MF et al. Permeability characteristics of the human small intestine. *J Clin Invest* 1965;44:1935-1944

5. Menzies IS: Transmucosal passage of inert molecules in health and disease. In: Skadhauge E, Heintze K, eds. Intestinal absorption and secretion. *Lancaster:MTP Press* 1984:527-543.

6. Uil JJ, van Elburg RM, van Overbeek FM et al. Clinical implications of the sugar absorption test: intestinal permeability test to assess mucosal barrier function. *Scand J Gastroenterol Suppl.* 1997;223:70-8.

CHAPTER 28

How to Prevent and Strengthen Leaky Gut Barrier

KEY POINTS

- Healthy feeding practices and exposure to farm animals in early life can reduce the risk of many chronic ailments.

- Supplements like turmeric, zinc, and glutamine can help strengthen the gut barrier.

Medicine is not a science; it is empiricism founded on a network of blunders.

—Emmet Densmore

The art and science of preventative and therapeutic aspects of leaky gut barrier is still in its infancy. However, we do have significant information from epidemiologic as well as laboratory studies that allow us to make prudent judgments as to what may be in our best health interests.

So let me just say the premier point at the outset. The best, the most prudent, and the easiest choice for leaky gut subjects is to eat all kinds of vegetables and fruit. The more diverse the choices of vegetables and fruits you make, the more likely it is that your gut will be healthy and strong.

LEAKY GUT PREVENTION

- Breast feed infants for the first six months of life. The intestinal barrier is immature in infancy allowing passage of large semi-digested dietary particles with potential for long-term allergies and autoimmune disease.

- Take kids to petting zoos and farms for outings especially during early childhood. Think of such trips not just for entertainment but as a part of disease prevention program.

- Avoid allergenic foods for two years especially cows' milk, chicken, eggs, peanuts, soy, and fish.

- Avoid nonsteroidal anti-inflammatory drugs like aspirin, Motrin®, Naproxen®, etc.

- Avoid the unnecessary use of antibiotics, especially in early life.

- Optimize coping mechanisms for stress.

USING SUPPLEMENTS TO STRENGTHEN LEAKY GUT

- Glutamine

- Turmeric or curcumin (Turmeric 2-3 g per day).

- Zinc 50 mg per day.

- Vitamin D 1000 to 2000 IU per day: vitamin D deficiency is widespread. Check levels!

PROBIOTICS ENHANCE BARRIER FUNCTION

- Reorient and revise the proteins protecting the *tight junctions* between the adjacent cells of the leaky gut barrier.

- Prevent barrier damage induced by excess oxidants and pro-inflammation chemicals in the body.

- Increase mucus lining of the gut wall preventing adhesion of bacteria to the wall and reducing risk of their passage across the leaky gut.

- Increase production of antibacterial compounds known as *defensins* which increases resistance of the intestinal wall to bacterial damage.

- Provide competition to the bad bacteria in the gut lumen thus preventing and/or displacing the attachment of bad bacteria to the gut wall. This reduces the risk of their passage across the gut wall and causing damage.

- Enhance healing of damaged cells comprising the gut barrier.

- Increase production of protective proteins by the cells.

- Prevent inflammation induced death of cells of gut barrier.

According to Dr. Lata and colleagues and as published in the *World Journal of Gastroenterology*, "Probiotics are able to decrease the permeability of intestinal wall and decrease bacterial translocation and endotoxemia...which is extremely important in preventing complications of liver cirrhosis and liver transplantation."

TREATMENT BASED ON UNDERLYING FACTORS

EXAMPLE OF TREATMENT OF SMALL INTESTINAL BACTERIAL OVERGROWTH

- Antibiotics especially gut selective antibiotics: Herbal antibacterial herbal products are also available e.g. Dysbiocide, FC Cidal, and ADP.

- Pro-motility agents that stimulate intestinal movements.

- Probiotics: Not all probiotics are created equal! Chapter 29: Probiotics and Prebiotics for Leaky Gut provides more details on probiotics for leaky gut.

STRENGTHEN BARRIER, TREAT LEAKY GUT!

- Remove the inciting cause.
- Make life style adjustments as appropriate.
  o Moderate exercise.
  o Maintain good orodental hygiene.
  o Regularize bowel habit to avoid constipation.
- Supplements like zinc, glutamine, turmeric, butyrate, aloe.
- Avoid refined sugar! Use healthier alternatives like stevia and honey.
- Elimination diet to exclude food triggers against allergy and inflammation.
- Acupuncture for slow gut to reduce stagnant bacteria in the bowels.

Traditional Chinese Medicine

Randomized controlled trials have shown that Dachengqi decoction decreases intestinal permeability and blood levels of bacterial toxin, along with reduced bacterial infections and multi-organ dysfunction in patients with acute pancreatitis, as compared to controls.

Bovine colostrum

Multiple studies have documented that bovine colostrum strengthens the intestinal barrier and reduces passage of intestinal bacteria across the gut wall into the body.

Glutamine

It is a useful nutrient for gut wall cells, as well as gut-associated immune cells. It promotes growth of intestinal cells with potential to strengthen gut barrier function. It maintains and/or restores the intestinal barrier and healthy balance of permeability in critically ill patients and improves their prognosis by reducing frequency of infections. It reduces chemotherapy-induced disruption of the gut barrier. Glutamine may sometimes have opposing effects depending on reasons underlying leaky gut.

- Glutamine deficit increases intestinal permeability in animals.
- Repletion of glutamine stores improves barrier in malnourished kids.
- Repletion helps barrier in critically sick patients and lowers frequency of infections.
- Glutamine lowers risk of allergies in low birth infants.

Taurine

Human milk is rich in the free amino-acid taurine. Relative taurine deficiency in early infancy has been implicated in adverse long-term neuro-developmental outcomes in preterm infants. As such, it is present as a supplement in formula milk and parenteral nutrition solutions for infants.

Enzyme-modified cheese

In vitro data suggests that enzyme-modified cheese inhibits passage of allergenic proteins across the gut wall into the body. Studies in rats with drug-induced intestinal damage confirm these beneficial effects on gut leakage.

Aged garlic extract

It prevents programmed cell death. It decreases disruption of the intestinal barrier and protects the intestine from damage due to cancer chemotherapy.

Calcium

Multiple controlled animal and human studies suggest that dietary calcium improves intestinal resistance and strengthens the intestinal barrier. Such an improvement of the barrier function is associated with improvement of colitis in animals.

NUTRITIONAL APPROACH TO STRENGTHEN BARRIER

Animal milk avoidance may help, since it alters the intestinal bacteria. Animal milk fat promotes inflammation in animal colitis. In contrast, fermented milk has beneficial effects against inflammation.

A nutritional approach to restore impaired intestinal barrier function and growth can be accomplished by using an adapted diet containing specific long-chain polyunsaturated fatty acids, prebiotics, and probiotics. Studies of stressed baby rats suggest that this diet reverses the negative effects of stress on the intestinal structure and body growth. Such data perhaps can be extrapolated to humans and evidence indicates biological plausibility.

A periodic detox program for clean gut to restore gut health helps many. I am biased against uncouth colonics. Rather, a cleaner practical and regular program of a juice/fast program is simpler and more practical and achieves desirable results. The detailed description of such a program is beyond the scope of this book. It is described in detail in the book, *Dr. M's Seven-X Plan for Digestive Health*.

> According to Drs. Rapin and Wiernperger from the University of Bergundy in France, "Intestinal permeability should be largely improved by dietary addition of compounds, such as glutamine or curcumin, which have the mechanistic potential to inhibit the inflammation and oxidative stress linked to tight junction openings."

Other potential therapeutic options that have shown beneficial experimental evidence include the following:

- Moxibustion
- Fish oil

- Butyrate
- Lactoferrin
- Glucagon-like peptide-2
- Flavonoids like Kaempferol (present in fruits, vegetables, tea) and quercetin
- Berberine
- Avoidance of high protein by otherwise healthy subjects

ROLE OF PHARMACEUTICAL INDUSTRY

Pharmaceutical companies are fast and furious pursuing a variety of strategies looking for ideal therapeutic options to strengthen leaky gut. Some of the medications currently used, e.g. anti-TNF medications used in inflammatory bowel disease, rheumatoid arthritis and psoriasis, are associated with decreased intestinal leakiness. A select listing of various options being investigated includes the following:

a. Growth factors like Teduglutide

b. Probiotics

c. Larazotide (blocks zonulin)

d. DA-6034 derived from flavonoids

e. DIMS-0150 or Kappaproct

f. HMPL-004, a natural product

REFERENCES

1. Catalito RM, Maggi CA, Giuliani S. Intestinal epithelial barrier dysfunction in disease and possible therapeutical interventions. *Curr Med Chem*. 2011;18(3):398-426.

2. Lu Z, Ding L, Lu Q, Chen YH. Claudins in intestines: Distribution and functional significance in health and diseases. *Tissue Barriers*. 2013 Jul1;1(3):e24978.

3. Li YC, Hsieh CC. Lactoferrin dampens high-fructose corn syrup-induced hepatic manifestations of the metabolic syndrome in a murine model. *PLoS One*. 2014 May9;9(5):e97341.

4. Wang B, Wu G, Zhou Z et al. Glutamine and intestinal barrier function. *Amino Acids*. 2014 Jun 26.

5. Price DB, Ackland ML, Burks W et al. Peanut allergens alter intestinal barrier permeability and tight junction localisation in Caco-2 cell cultures. *Cell Physiol Biochem*. 2014 May 23;33(6):1758-1777.

CHAPTER 29

Probiotics and Prebiotics for Leaky Gut

KEY POINTS

- Probiotics alter the bacterial balance only temporarily. Hence, they have to be taken consistently over the long-term for health benefits.

- All probiotics are not equal in efficacy for all conditions.

A healthy gut has at least 90% of good bacteria or normal healthy inhabitants. In unhealthy states, the number is down and the virulence of bad bacteria is relatively higher.

A healthy dose of the probiotic bacteria can help tilt the balance. Most but not all probiotics are bacteria. *Saccharomyces boulardii* is an example of a popular probiotic fungus.

Use of foods like yogurt with live cultures, kimchi, sauerkraut, miso, kombucha, and kefir containing probiotics should be encouraged in general. While cow's milk can have lot of issues related to it, a fermented product is a different story altogether.

Please note that probiotic food products from different sources do not contain the same types or amounts of probiotics. This is particularly true for yogurts that may or may not have live cultures.

Some yogurt brands may just have two standard bacteria strains in limited amounts while other brands may have multiple probiotic strains in much higher numbers to really provide the extra-solid punch.

ALL PROBIOTICS ARE *NOT* CREATED SIMILAR OR EQUAL

Examples of probiotics that strengthen gut barrier

- VSL#3

- L. rhamnosus Gorbach-Goldin

- Lactobacillus plantarum 299v

- Lactobacillus johnsonii

- PB6 (Bacillus subtilis)

- Bifidobacterium adolescentis

- Bifidobacter lactis

- Saccharomyces boulardii

- Combination of Lactobacillus plantarum CGMCC No. 1258, Lactobacillus acidophilus LA-11, and Bifido-bacterium longum BL-88

- Combination of Streptococcus thermophilus, Lactobacillus bulgaricus, Lactobacillus acidophilus, and Bifidobacterium Longum

- Lactobacillus rhamnosus 19070-2 and L. reuteri DSM 12246

Unless a particular bacterial strain and formulation has been shown to be helpful in a particular condition, the following general principles may be used when buying a probiotic product at a store.

Study the fine print on the label wisely

The probiotic formulation should state the genus, species, and preferably the strain of the probiotic. Just genus and species may not always be enough since different strains can have different effects.

Type and number of bacteria is important

Pay careful attention to the number of organisms or CFUs contained in a single formulation.

Unless a particular strain has been shown to be of benefit, one should pick a formulation with multiple types of bacteria, in my opinion at least 4 types. Others have argued for at least 7 types of probiotic strains. Pay particular attention to whether those strains have been shown to be of benefit in studies.

There is strength in numbers

There should be at least 5 if not 10 billion bacteria or CFUs in the formulation. The higher the number, the more they are likely to be able to survive stomach acid and digestive juices and reach the colon in greater numbers.

Third party certifications

It is better to buy a product that has been certified by an independent third party. Studies have shown that many formulations don't contain the type or number of bacteria (CFUs) that the label claims.

The Food and Drug Administration (FDA) is generally not involved in regulation of probiotics unless claims of healing against particular sickness are made. VSL#3 is a unique example of a probiotic formulation that is FDA regulated.

IMPORTANCE OF PREBIOTICS

Undigested carbohydrates, usually fiber, act as food for the gut wall. They potentiate the growth of healthy gut bacteria as well healthy effects of probiotics.

FIBER-FREE DIET MAKES GUT LEAKY

The intestines of animals fed a fiber-free diet are leakier than those fed fiber. The American diet sorely lacks in fiber. We need about 25-35g of fiber daily. Fiber consumed should include both the soluble and insoluble kind. Half of your plate in each meal should be fruit and vegetables. Use vegetables of different colors to complement their beneficial impact.

EXAMPLES OF NATURALLY DELICIOUS PREBIOTICS

- Garlic
- Leek
- Ginger
- Artichokes
- Bananas
- Watermelon
- Honey

Commercial formulations of prebiotics are also available on market.

> Green banana and pectin fibers reduce intestinal permeability and improve diarrhea in kids in developing countries.

REFERENCES

1. Sanders ME, Lenoir-Wijnkoop I, Salminen S et al. Probiotics and prebiotics: prospects for public health and nutritional recommendations. *Ann N Y Acad Sci*. 2014 Feb; 1309:19-29.

2. Mackowiak PA. Recycling Metchnikoff: Probiotics, the Intestinal Microbiome and the Quest for Long Life. *Front Public Health*. 2013 Nov 13; 1:52.

3. Petschow B, Doré J, Hibberd P et al. Probiotics, prebiotics, and the host microbiome: the science of translation. *Ann N Y Acad Sci.* 2013 Dec; 1306:1-17.

4. Saulnier DM, Ringel Y, Heyman MB et al. The intestinal microbiome, probiotics and prebiotics in neurogastroenterology. *Gut Microbes.* 2013 Jan-Feb; 4(1):17-27.

CHAPTER 30

Holistic Gut-Venture Beyond Leaky Barrier

KEY POINTS

- The gut is a very complex organ with built in redundancies. A focus solely on "leaky gut" may not be sufficient in some cases.

- A comprehensive gut healing program is important but should always be undertaken in consultation with your physician.

THE BIG PICTURE

Referring you to the initial chapters, let us not forget the big picture. The gut is a very complex organ with multiple interactions and redundancies built in.

Such a situation can sometimes resist isolated and focused treatment strategies. As such, a comprehensive gut-fixing program may sometimes be needed, especially in difficult cases. Various experts have come up with and written about their recommended strategies.

ONE SIZE DOES NOT FIT ALL

An ideal gut-fixing digestive health program would allow you to tailor it according to your bodily needs and constitution. After all, one size does not fit all.

Take an example of 100 persons falling from their bikes during a race. Even though the situation may occur under similar circumstances of speed, road conditions, and weather, etc., the extent of injuries is likely to be different.

While some may just have superficial injuries or even a simple fracture, a few may have multiple and compound fractures and even rupture of internal organs.

Obviously, the patients with simple injuries could just be treated in the ER and released; some may need a brace or a cast for a simple fracture, whereas a few may need surgery and internal fixation of the bones as well as treatment of other injuries.

The depth and breadth of diversity of treatment of illness related to leaky gut may likewise occur.

COMPLEX SITUATIONS REQUIRE COMPREHENSIVE STRATEGY

Opinions vary on what is the best approach. I am biased in favor of the comprehensive and holistic strategy outlined in my book *Dr. M's Seven-X Plan for Digestive Health.*

The *Seven-X Plan* provides an all-embracing approach that includes nutritional therapy and healing of dysbiosis. Uncontrolled inflammation and oxidative stress needs to be countered. For example, a multivitamin, multi-mineral supplement improves symptoms of chronic fatigue syndrome, possibly related to boosting antioxidant defenses.

Sometimes, the answer lies not in what you should take, rather in what you should avoid. A pharmaceutical pill should not be ideal answer to all of nature's problems. Do you need to be on an elimination diet? If so, what kind of diet? Paleo? Gluten free? Low FODMAP? Do you understand the how, what and why of these exclusion diets?

Furthermore, is cow's milk good or bad? Is vegetarianism healthy or harmful for you?

A colon cleanse and detox may be helpful but going through uncouth colonics may not be the best or the easiest answer. *Dr. M's Seven-X Plan* also provides a detailed weekly and monthly juice/fast program that is healthy, easier to accomplish, and is more likely to be effective in keeping the body rejuvenated in a sustained fashion.

While *Dr. M's Seven-X Plan* reflects my personal bias, there may be other programs that may be better suited to your individual needs. You and your health care provider are the best judge of your situation as to what would work best for you.

DR. M'S CLOSING THOUGHTS

Some would argue that the issue of "leaky gut syndrome" has not been categorically settled in the medical literature; that data linking it to diseases is circumstantial and sometimes preliminary and conflicting.

They may be correct, but isn't that always the case about medical science which is always dynamic and fluid, wherein concepts get outdated within a few years of being touted as "state of the art?"

In fact, it is entirely possible that the cutting edge treatment you have been prescribed for your condition may actually represent an outdated treatment of the future.

THE CHOICE IS YOURS

The question before you is simple. After reading this book and hopefully doing some more research on your own, including checking out the references provided, are you convinced that leaky gut may be, just may be, an underlying factor for your chronic difficult to treat ailment?

Can you afford to continue to suffer illness that persists despite usual medical treatment? Are you sure if the issue of leaky gut will be absolutely settled even during our lifetime? Or should you try some additional measures, not in lieu of, but as adjunct in consultation with your physician?

True health reform begins with you. A day without health is another day of suffering.

I agree wholeheartedly that the relationship between leaky gut and sickness is ripe for further exploration. I am also convinced that, depending upon clinical context, it is prudent to adopt a strategy against leaky gut by implementing measures to strengthen the intestinal barrier, including a "leaky-gut diet." This should, however, always be undertaken in conjunction with and after discussion with your physician. No book can serve as a substitute for the knowledge and wisdom of your physician who knows you and your needs the best!

Health is wealth.

May God bless you and all those around you with the best of health.

A personal note from Dr. Minocha

I truly appreciate you taking the time to read my thoughts on leaky gut. If you liked the book, I would be extremely grateful if you would please show your love and support by writing an honest review for it at the amazon.com and goodreads.com websites.

Tell the potential readers what you liked about the book and what you plan to do with the information. Your review would also help in my mission to share knowledge and promote health.

Thanks a million!

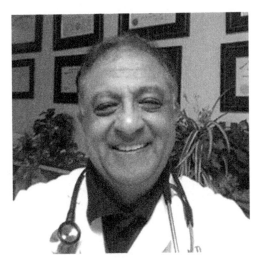

Anil Minocha MD

PS: I would love to connect with you on Facebook@doctoranil and Twitter@dranilminocha.

Dedication

This book is dedicated to my family: my loving parents Ram and Kamla, my siblings Kamal, Vimal and Rina, and the light of my life Geeta. Without their unconditional love and support, this book would not have been possible.

Praise for
"Dr. M's Seven-X Plan for Digestive Health"

"If you are looking for a holistic whole-body solution to your digestive ailments, then this is the book for you! "

— Dr. Robynne Chutkan, author of *Gutbliss*

"A treasure trove of key information on probiotics, intestinal infections and everything you ever could want to know about the digestive system."

— Chris Adamec, co-author of *Fibromyalgia for Dummies*

"In particular, I found the information on the role of bacteria is in gut health as well as GI disease and dysfunction, a subject that often leaves many healthcare providers scratching their heads, very helpful and his description of his practical Seven-X Plan is easy to understand and follow."

— Jill Sklar, author of The First Year: Crohn's Disease and Ulcerative Colitis.

"If the proverbial 'cast iron' describes only other people's stomachs, you'll be fascinated by this accessible and infinitely helpful guide to your own GI system and how to keep it healthy -- information that just might cause you to start feeling good all over."

— Victoria Moran, author of *Main Street Vegan*

Other Books by Dr. Minocha

Dr. M's Seven-X Plan for Digestive Health

A Guide to Alternative System and the Digestive System

Encyclopedia of Digestive System and Digestive Disorders

Handbook of Digestive Diseases

Natural Stomach Care (2003)

CPSIA information can be obtained
at www.ICGtesting.com
Printed in the USA
LVOW04s1713261016
510385LV00011B/1187/P